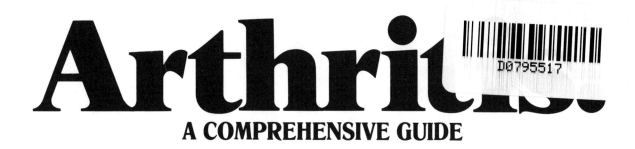

Arthritis

A COMPREHENSIVE GUIDE

Arthritis.

A COMPREHENSIVE GUIDE

James F. Fries, M.D.

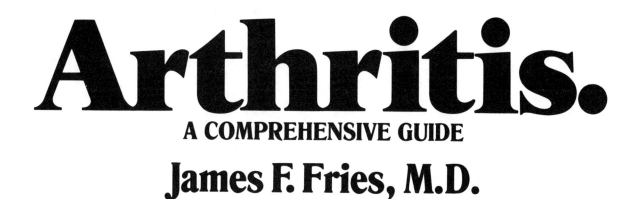

ADDISON-WESLEY PUBLISHING COMPANY

READING, MASSACHUSETTS • MENLO PARK, CALIFORNIA
LONDON • AMSTERDAM • DON MILLS, ONTARIO • SYDNEY

Library of Congress Cataloging in Publication Data

Fries, James F
  Arthritis.

  Bibliography: p.
  Includes index.
  1. Arthritis. I. Title. [DNLM: 1. Arthritis--
Popular works. WE344 F912a]
RC933.F75   616.7'2   79-50868
ISBN 0-201-02725-9

Fourth Printing, April 1982

ISBN 0-201-02725-9-H
      0-201-02726-7-P
DEFGHIJKLM-DO-898765432

To Sarah,
with my love

Preface

Three new concepts provide the intellectual framework for this book.

First, it is now known to be crucial that each individual assume greater personal responsibility for his or her own health, that the medical consumer has a right to know, and that dependable information sources are needed.

Second, a revolution in medical thinking has occurred; it is now known that the body lasts longer when it is used and ages more rapidly with disuse. This concept usually has been emphasized for cardiac and muscular fitness; it holds to a surprising degree for the joints.

Third, it is now recognized that withdrawal from social interaction, from new experiences, and from the exercise of personal autonomy all accelerate the aging process. Arthritis is in many ways a physical parallel to psychological aging; it is an allegory for the aging process. When arthritis is incorrectly regarded as an unsolvable problem of increasing pain and decreasing function, it can become a reason for retreat from independent life. The therapeutic response to arthritis thus extends far beyond the joints; the successful response to musculoskeletal pain must be reaffirmation of life rather than its rejection.

Among those to whom I am indebted for understanding of these concepts are: Paul Baltes, James Birren, John Bunker, Lionel Cosin, Rene Dubos, Alain Enthoven, Jack Farquhar, Victor Fuchs, Halsted Holman, John Knowles, Ralph Paffenbarger, Matilda Riley, and Martin Seligman.

I am also indebted to the many patients, physicians, and patient educators who contributed experiences and perspective to the development of this manuscript. Their suggestions have resulted in hundreds of specific additions and changes. Any remaining deficiencies are my responsibility. I particularly acknowledge the contributions of:

Dr. Rodney Bluestone, Dr. Jack Boyer, Dr. Melvin Britton, Dr. Andrei Calin, Marie Cascio, Dr. Stephen Cole, Dr. George Ehrlich, Dr. Wallace Epstein, Lois Fleming, Dr. Bevra Hahn, Dr. Evelyn Hess, Dr. L. A. Healey, Dr. William Lages, Dr. Michael Lockshin, Kate Lorig, R.N., Dr. Dennis McShane, Dr. Donald Mitchell, Janice Pigg, R.N., Gene Fauro Pratt, Carol Rice, O.T., Irene Seligman, Dee Simpson, Patricia Spitz, R.N., Annette Swezey, M.P.H., Dr. Cody Wasner, Dr. Gordon Williams.

Manuscript preparation would not have been possible without long hours of effort by Sharon Joseph. Scip Wylbur typed and retyped the manuscript tirelessly. My wife, Sarah, and my children, Elizabeth and Gregory, gracefully endured my preoccupations during the endeavor.

The communication techniques developed for *Take Care of Yourself* and used again in *Taking Care of Your Child* are employed in this volume. I hope that they succeed in clarifying this neglected and complicated subject. If so, it is due in large part to my collaborations with Dr. Donald Vickery and with the editorial staff at Addison-Wesley.

Stanford, California   J. F. F.
April 1979

Contents

PART II   MANAGING YOUR ARTHRITIS

7
DUCK THAT QUACK   143

8
SAVING MONEY SAFELY   149

9
PREVENTING ARTHRITIS   155

PART III   SOLVING PROBLEMS WITH ARTHRITIS

10
GENERAL PROBLEMS   161

11
PROBLEMS WITH PAIN   175

PART IV   ADDITIONAL INFORMATION

PART

I

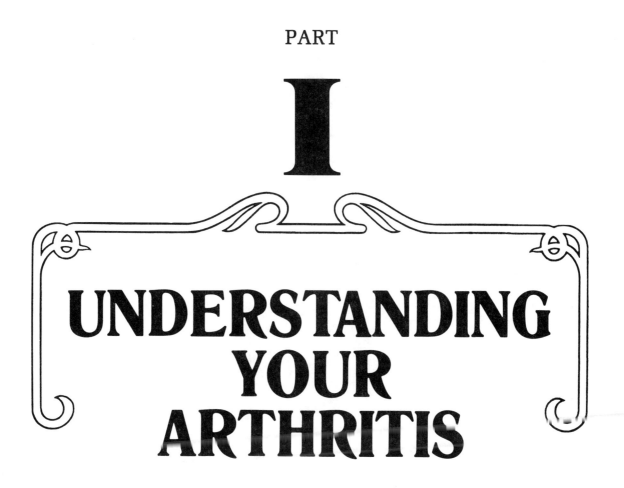

UNDERSTANDING YOUR ARTHRITIS

1

Defeating Arthritis

You have much more control over your arthritis or rheumatism than you may think. You do not have to be a victim of these common medical problems. Rather, you can defeat them, and lead a full, normal life. To do this, you need to know something about arthritis. You need to know how to prevent damage to joint tissues. And you need to know how to get relief when special problems arise. In short, you need to know what is happening in your body and what you can do about it.

For some curious reason, the idea lingers that "nothing can be done for arthritis." The very opposite is true. Probably more progress has been made in the fight against arthritis than in the struggle against our other major diseases—cancer, heart disease, and diabetes. You can benefit from these advances.

The battle against certain forms of arthritis is nearly won. Rheumatoid arthritis, the most common major arthritis, is under attack from a number of promising new treatments. Gout, a major disease of the past, now yields readily to treatment. Systemic lupus erythematosus, once a mysterious and very serious ailment, is now successfully managed in almost every case. New surgical advances, such as joint replacement, often prove dramatically helpful. Genetic factors have been identified for many kinds of arthritis, and our understanding of the molecular basis for joint disease is increasing rapidly.

As arthritis has become better understood, its complexity has become more apparent. Over one hundred different kinds of arthritis have now been identified. Every kind of arthritis, and ultimately every patient, is different. For treatment to be effective, it is essential to find the treatment most suitable for the individual under care. Knowledge of how to accurately match treatment to patient is not yet complete, and many patients undergo several kinds of treatment before the right one is found. If you know about recent advances in the field and the problems yet to be solved, you can help with your own treatment program.

Successfully managing your arthritis depends on you as much as on your doctor. Your decisions are ultimately the most important. You decide:

- How much activity to undertake

- Whether to see the doctor, and when

- What kind of doctor to see

- When to ask for a second opinion

- Whether to accept the medical advice offered

- Whether to follow a treatment program carefully

- Whether to seek a quack cure or to believe a sensational tabloid story

Ultimately, you decide how much you weigh, what you think of yourself, and what you want to do with your life. Your doctor will be a great help to you. But you have to make the decisions and carry them out.

Think of this book as a series of conversations with your doctor about your problems. We who treat patients with arthritis have had these conversations hundreds of times. But sometimes the demands of office or clinic don't give us enough time for in-depth discussion. Sometimes the conversation is forgotten by the patient or only parts of it are remembered. Often, the patient thinks of new questions after the visit is over. Here you can read and reread the discussion in full, and you can refer to pertinent sections to refresh your understanding when a particular problem arises.

An "arthritis victim" is someone who has been defeated by arthritis. Instead, your goal is to come out on top—to defeat your arthritis. Your arthritis can be helped. In some cases, it can be cured. Even when it cannot be cured totally, your life can be full and complete. You can be independent and happy. This book is about resources: medical resources, community resources, and most importantly your own resources. You aren't blind, your heart works fine, your mind is alert. This book is about how to defeat the pains and stiffness in your body.

IF YOU HAVE PAIN, DO YOU HAVE ARTHRITIS?

In the truest sense of the word, most "arthritis" is not really arthritis at all! Doctors use the term *arthritis* differently than do patients. The *arth* part of the word means "joint"—not muscle, tendon, ligament, or bone. The *itis* part means "inflamed." Thus, true arthritis affects the joints, and the inflamed joints are red, warm, swollen, or tender when squeezed. If you do not have any of these symptoms, then you do not have arthritis in the true sense of the term.

However, in common usage, the term *arthritis* refers to almost any painful condition of the muscles or the skeletal system. *Rheumatism* is an imprecise term that includes not only problems with the joints, but any problems affecting the body's musculoskeletal system. In this book, we have taken a very broad view of what constitutes arthritis and rheumatism, and you will find descriptions and treatments for all major problems affecting the muscles, joints, or the areas around the joints—from rheumatoid arthritis to sciatica to bursitis.

HOW COMMON IS ARTHRITIS?

In the United States, seventy-five million people experience some symptoms in their joints and muscles from time to time. Twenty-two million have moderate problems from their arthritis, and nearly three million Americans are severely affected. Thus, we can talk about arthritis either as a national problem that, although very common, is usually relatively mild or as an extremely severe problem that affects a smaller number of people. Whichever way you look at it, arthritis and rheumatism cause more work loss, more pain, and more poor functioning in daily life than does any other kind of human illness. But arthritis can be prevented in many cases and effective treatment is available for all forms of these diseases.

DO YOU NEED A DOCTOR?

Few of us go even a single year without some episode of pain or stiffness. So, we have to be able to decide when a condition requires the care of a physician and when we can take care of it ourselves. The decision chart presented here will help you answer this general question. If you have a specific problem listed in Part III, refer to that particular decision chart for assistance in deciding whether to see the doctor.

Only rarely does a patient with muscle or joint pain need a physician immediately. Home treatment and patience will resolve most problems. It is important to remember that, for most problems involving the musculoskeletal system, the natural healing process requires two to six weeks. Drugs do not accelerate this natural healing process. For most problems, therefore, a period of watchful waiting is the most important treatment.

The relative emergencies are infection, nerve damage, fractures near a joint, and gout. In the first three, serious damage may result if the joint is neglected; in the fourth, the pain is so intense that immediate help is needed. "Immediate" means at least to call the doctor today. Most complications of arthritis occur slowly and are more easily prevented than corrected. A persistent musculoskeletal problem always should be brought to the attention of a physician, but allow "tincture of time" to sort out trivial injuries or strains from more significant conditions. Remember that arthritis results in more lost work days and more sickness than does any other kind of disease—it

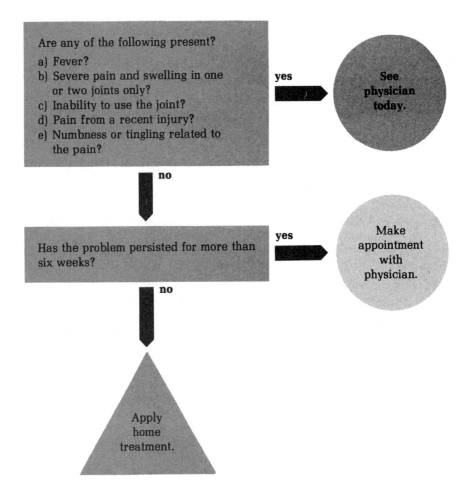

Are any of the following present?
a) Fever?
b) Severe pain and swelling in one
   or two joints only?
c) Inability to use the joint?
d) Pain from a recent injury?
e) Numbness or tingling related to
   the pain?

yes → **See physician today.**

no

Has the problem persisted for more than six weeks?

yes → Make appointment with physician.

no

Apply home treatment.

must be managed correctly and with care. Not too much concern, but not too little either.

Run your finger down the decision chart. Fever, usually over 100°F, indicates the possibility of infection or a severe form of arthritis. Surprisingly, arthritis affecting only a few joints is more urgent than arthritis affecting many joints. Both gout and infection usually involve only one or two joints. If the joint can't be used, it may be significantly injured and it is in danger of permanent stiffness. Again, immediate attention is required. And, if the pain comes from an injury that might have caused a broken bone, see a physician. If pain from the back runs down the side of the leg to the foot, if there is numbness or tingling in the fingers of the hand, or if there is an area of numbness on the head when you move your neck, there may be nerve damage. Any such symptoms should be brought to the attention of a doctor immediately.

Fortunately, arthritis pains aren't very often associated with any of those things. More frequently, the problem will simply go away slowly over several weeks. In the instances when it persists for more than six weeks, it is again wise to consult a doctor.

If you are going to wait six weeks, what can you do at home? Rest, warmth, and minor pain medication make up the initial home treatment. Remember that the purpose of pain is not to make us miserable, but to prevent us from injuring ourselves. If a joint is painful when you move it, your body is telling you to rest that part. Using too much pain medication can result in overuse of an inflamed joint and can cause additional damage. So, keep the pain relief mild and simple. Aspirin—two tablets four times a day—or acetaminophen (Tylenol) in the same dosage is often satisfactory. Aspirin, as we discuss later, is a marvelously powerful drug for the treatment of arthritis when taken in much higher doses. But use of aspirin as a powerful anti-inflammatory drug should seldom be started in the first six weeks of a problem.

What else can you do for yourself? There are many other measures you can take. Read about them in the remainder of Parts I and II and under the heading of your particular problems in Part III.

Time is the only known cure for most problems that affect the musculoskeletal system. When you develop a new complaint, you must use time to separate the trivial from the serious. Luckily, the trivial outnumbers the serious by at least twenty to one. In most instances, the body's repair process involves resting the affected part by use of the pain mechanism and by bringing in new materials with which to reconstruct the injured area. Through most of this book, we will be focusing on the few percent of musculoskeletal problems that continue, problems that may result in significant health difficulties.

HOW TO USE THIS BOOK

This book can be a great help to you if used correctly. More arthritis information is provided here than has previously been publicly available. But this book is not a doctor. It will help you understand your arthritis and your doctor's treatments, and it may provide you with more detailed explanations than your doctor has time to give. The medical content of this book has been reviewed by many physicians expert in the care of patients with arthritis. I have indicated general consensus on a particular point by using "we"; if my opinion might differ from those of some of my colleagues, I have used "I" to indicate the source.

All serious forms of arthritis require the care of a physician. In an individual case, the recommendations given in this book may not be just right. So, if you are under the care of a physician and receive advice contrary to this book, follow the physician's advice; the individual characteristics of your case can then be taken into account.

There are many different kinds of arthritis, and you will usually be bothered by only one. There are also many drugs that may be useful, many tests that may be performed, and many operations that might be needed. You will need only a few. This book is organized to guide you to the sections that pertain to you, skipping over those that do not apply.

Read what you need. Next month or next year you may need to refer to some different sections.

There are three important steps that you can take toward defeating your arthritis, and this book is organized around them:

1. With Part I of this book, **you can identify what kind of arthritis you have** and choose the best treatment and medication to defeat it. First, use the simple charts at the beginning of Chapter 2 to identify your category of arthritis. Each of the nine categories in the rest of the chapter includes detailed discussions on specific types of arthritis. These discussions will lead you to pertinent information on the best treatment, medication, and tests for your type of arthritis.

2. Part II of this book has important information on **managing your arthritis,** including: treatments (Chapter 3), medications (Chapter 4), surgery (Chapter 5), tests (Chapter 6), avoiding quack treatments (Chapter 7), saving money (Chapter 8), and preventing arthritis (Chapter 9).

3. Part III is designed to help you **cope with everyday problems** with pain, with medication side effects, with getting around, with sex, and with your work. Look up your specific problem in the Table of Contents. The charts in this section of the book will help you decide whether you can treat yourself at home or whether you need to see a doctor or other health professional.

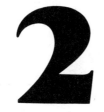

What Kind of Arthritis Do You Have?

THE EIGHT MAJOR CATEGORIES

There are 109 kinds of arthritis currently known. They range from rare to common and from trivial to serious. Unfortunately, too many people think of arthritis as a single disease. Selecting the treatment that will help you the most depends on the type of arthritis active in your body.

You can understand the process that's causing your pain or stiffness without reading about 109 diseases or going to medical school. Arthritis has only eight major categories, and this chapter tells you about them.

Some arthritis diagnoses can be difficult for even the most skilled physicians and may require laboratory tests and X-rays that are not available to you. Your doctor is more experienced than you are at making the observations that help in the diagnosis. Any person with arthritis who meets the criteria noted earlier in Chapter 1 or has pain for longer than six weeks should be seen by a physician. So, be sure you have a doctor.

You can help your doctor a great deal by understanding what is happening in your body and what can be done about it. Identify your arthritis category. This will help you better understand why you are experiencing certain symptoms. But leave the diagnosis to your doctor.

The accompanying diagram shows a joint. The joint is faced with a layer of *cartilage* (or gristle) on each side. The joint membrane, called the *synovial membrane*, surrounds the joint space and provides lubricating fluid for the cartilage surfaces. Fibrous tissue (the *joint capsule*) connects the bones and gives stability to the joint. Muscles taper down into tendon *leaders* and attach to the bone, usually just above or just below a joint. In some parts of the body, *bursae* lie between two muscles (or between muscles and tendons) to lubricate body tissues that must move across each other.

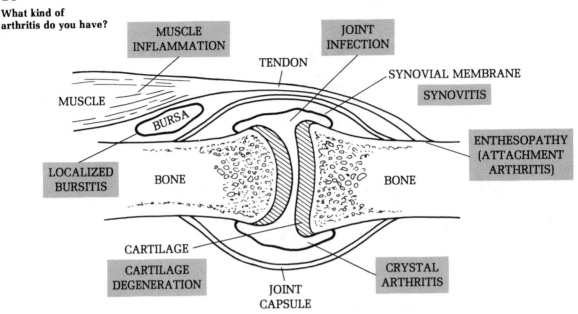

That's the anatomy lesson. The joint is remarkably well engineered. The cartilage is spongy and absorbs shock, the action is self-lubricating, and the mechanism is self-healing following injury. Good design. Now that you know the anatomy, you also know the eight categories! Each category of arthritis attacks a different body structure.

The accompanying table summarizes the eight categories in a simple way. There are exceptions to these rules, but we will get to those later. Notice that each category has a different basic problem and a different basic treatment. There is a ninth category, "Not Quite Arthritis," which is a little more complicated and is described later in this chapter.

The first category is **synovitis**. This big word simply means that the synovial membrane, which creates the lubricating fluid for the joint, is inflamed. Inflammation makes it red, warm, tender, or swollen. The major synovitis is called *rheumatoid arthritis*, or *RA*; it can occur at any age and it affects mostly women. Treatment is different for every individual, but a typically effective treatment is aspirin in high doses.

The second category I have named **attachment arthritis**. This term is a new one and your doctor may not be familiar with it, I have used it to help you understand the process. Doctors often call this disease process **enthesopathy**, but people have trouble understanding this word. Here, the primary inflammation is not in the joint membrane but occurs where the ligaments and tendons attach to the bone. This condition affects men more often than women and usually begins between age 15 and age 40. *Ankylosing spondylitis* (*AS* or *poker spine*) is the most common attachment arthritis.

Crystal arthritis is sometimes called **microcrystalline** by physicians, because the crystals are very small. They form in the joint space itself. As the body tries to remove the crystals, a painful inflammation occurs. The most dramatic example of this process is *gout*. These conditions affect men more frequently than women and usually begin in middle life or later.

Joint infections make up the fourth category. Here, there are bacteria in the joint fluid. These infections can occur at any age and in either sex; young persons are most frequently infected with the *gonococcal* (gc) bacterium while older individuals frequently have the *staphylococcus* germ.

Cartilage degeneration is the fifth category. The cartilage that faces the joints can wear down with age. This forms the "wear and tear" arthritis we call *osteoarthritis* or *osteoarthrosis*. It usually is noticed in middle life or later and is so common that all of us, if we live long enough, will experience some features of it.

The sixth category is **muscle inflammation**. This problem isn't really in the joint at all. However, many patients complaining of arthritis actually have problems in the muscles or other tissues. These diseases are more unusual and can affect either sex at any age.

THE ARTHRITIS CATEGORIES

Category	What's happening?	Who gets it?	Most typical diseases in this category	Typical treatment
Synovitis	Inflamed membrane of the joint	Any age, mostly women	Rheumatoid arthritis	Aspirin, high dose
Attachment arthritis (enthesopathy)	Inflamed ligament attachment to bone	Mostly men, onset age 15–40	Ankylosing spondylitis	Indomethacin, Phenylbutazone
Crystal arthritis	Chemical crystals in the joint fluid	Mostly men, onset age 35–90	Gout	Colchicine Allopurinol
Joint infection	Bacteria in the joint fluid	Any age, either sex	Staphylococcus, gonococcus	Antibiotics
Cartilage degeneration	Breakdown of joint cartilage	Either sex, age 45–90	Osteoarthrosis, osteoarthritis	Aspirin, low dose
Muscle inflammation	Inflamed muscle tissues	Either sex, any age	Polymyalgia rheumatica, polymyositis	Prednisone
Local conditions	Local injury	Either sex, any age	Low back strain, tennis elbow, frozen shoulder	Local measures
General conditions	Poorly defined	Either sex, any age	Fibrositis	Exercise

Local conditions make up the seventh category. These are not really diseases. For the most part, local problems result from a local irritation or injury. The back has suffered a strain or a sprain, there is pull of the ligament around the elbow as a result of playing tennis, or some other minor accident, often unnoticed, has led to pain in a single region of the body. If you treat these conditions carefully, they usually aren't too much of a problem.

The eighth category is termed **general conditions**. These conditions are poorly understood, but involve aching and stiffness throughout the body. These difficulties can occur in either sex and at any age, but are rather more common in the thirties, forties, and early fifties than at other ages. Doctors are just beginning to recognize some of the different conditions within this group and to devise effective treatments for them.

The accompanying decision chart will help you quickly determine your arthritis category. This chart will give you the correct category about 90 percent of the time, and if you check your result with "The Features of Arthritis Categories" table and with the discussion in the appropriate section of this chapter, you are unlikely to be misled. If your doctor has told you what your diagnosis is, look it up in the index, then go directly to the pertinent discussion.

Let's look at the reasons for the questions posed in the decision chart. How many parts of the body hurt? Infections, crystal arthritis, and local conditions usually affect only one part of the body, and synovitis and cartilage degeneration sometimes affect only one part. Distinction between these takes place as we move across the chart, responding to successive questions.

Is a joint warm, swollen, or tender? Remember that pain in the muscles and joints is not the same as true arthritis, which by definition means "inflamed joint tissues." If there is not true arthritis, by definition we have a "local condition." With an injury, a local condition is again likely. Arthritis in a child (under 16) may be the synovitis of juvenile rheumatoid arthritis or acute rheumatic fever. If fever is present in an adult, we have a problem with a "single hot joint" in which infection must be suspected. If the pain persists for over two weeks, cartilage degeneration in a single joint, perhaps a knee, is likely; rarely it may be a synovitis. The single hot joint without any fever or injury is likely to be a crystal arthritis.

Suppose that several parts of the body hurt. Then, we use the left side of the decision chart. If low back pain or heel pain is present, the problem is likely to be an attachment arthritis. If the low back hasn't been affected, the question is whether there are obvious signs of inflammation in a joint. If so, then it is most likely a synovitis. If not, are there signs of inflammation in the muscles? If all answers are no, then it is most likely a generalized condition. Synovitis usually is associated with discomfort in the morning, while cartilage degeneration leads to more discomfort later in the day; the morning stiffness frequenlty lasts 30 minutes or longer.

Synovitis usually involves both sides of the body relatively equally, involves a different pattern of joints, and is more "boggy" to the touch over

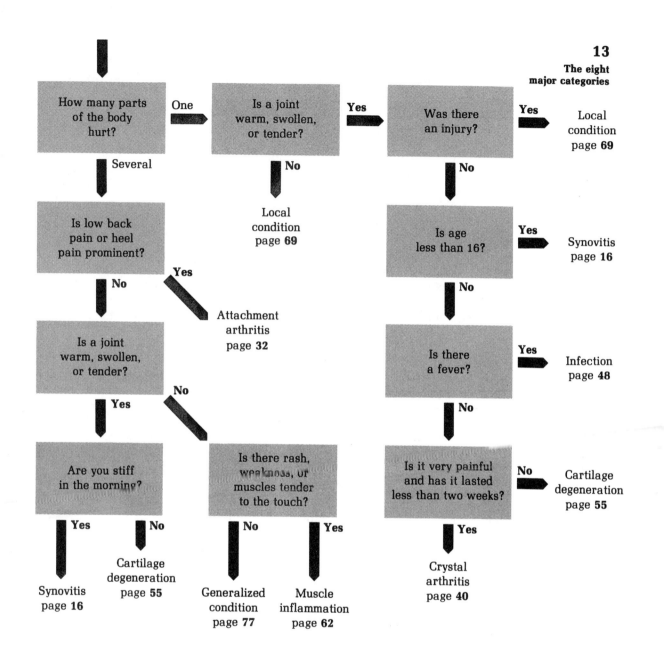

the joint, but these distinctions are often difficult to make, even for the doctor. Your doctor will use a slightly different logic to determine the category of your arthritis, but this decision chart has been constructed using questions you can answer yourself.

After you have determined a category, check the table, "Features of Arthritis Categories," to see if the category makes sense for your arthritis.

The severity of the inflammation is greatest with crystal arthritis or with infection of the joint. Such joints can be exquisitely painful and very warm to the touch. With synovitis, the joint inflammation is usually pretty obvious but is not quite as striking. Crystal arthritis and joint infection come on more rapidly than do the other conditions; this is what is meant by "acute." Other problems typically develop over a period of days or weeks, whereas these two problems may come on within hours.

Each of the categories typically attacks different parts of the body. Synovitis affects the knuckles, wrists, and knees. Attachment arthritis affects the low back and sometimes the heels. Crystal arthritis usually affects a knee, an ankle, or the base of the great toe. Joint infection involves most commonly a knee or other large joints. Cartilage degeneration tends to affect the finger joints at the end of the finger; these joints are often spared in a synovitis. The neck can be involved by degenerative arthritis, as can the low back or the weight-bearing joints of the legs. Muscle inflammation involves the muscles and usually spares the joints themselves. Local conditions affect only a single region and general conditions tend to be very poorly described by the patient, who often isn't sure exactly where the pain and discomfort are coming from.

FEATURES OF ARTHRITIS CATEGORIES

Category	Came on fast?	Typical place affected?	Only one part of the body?	Morning stiffness?	Fever?
Synovitis	No	Fingers, wrists, knees	Usually many	Marked	Rare
Attachment arthritis (enthesopathy)	No	Low back, heels	Usually several	Some	No
Crystal arthritis	Yes	Knee, ankle, great toe	Yes	No	No
Joint infection	Yes	Knee, hip, shoulder	Yes	No	Yes
Cartilage degeneration	No	End finger joints, hips, knees, neck, low back	Usually	No	No
Muscle inflammation	No	Muscles, not joints	No	Some	Rare
Local conditions	Yes	Elbow, shoulder, low back	Yes	No	No
General conditions	No	All over	No	No	No

All right, you know your category and can understand generally what is happening to you. Now go to the appropriate section of this chapter and read in detail about the diseases that make up your category. The following list will help you quickly locate the section of interest.

- **Synovitis** (page 16): rheumatoid arthritis, juvenile arthritis, lupus (SLE), psoriatic arthritis

- **Attachment arthritis** (page 32): ankylosng spondylitis (AS), Reiter's syndrome

- **Crystal arthritis** (page 40): gout, pseudogout

- **Joint infection** (page 48): staph, GC, tuberculosis

- **Cartilage degeneration** (page 55): osteoarthritis, Charcot joints

- **Muscle inflammation** (page 62): polymyositis (PM), dermatomyositis (DM), polymyalgia rheumatica (PMR)

- **Local conditions** (page 69): tennis elbow, bursitis, back strain, lumbar disks

- **General conditions** (page 77): fibrositis, psychosomatic conditions, depression

Synovitis:

Inflammation of the Joint Membrane

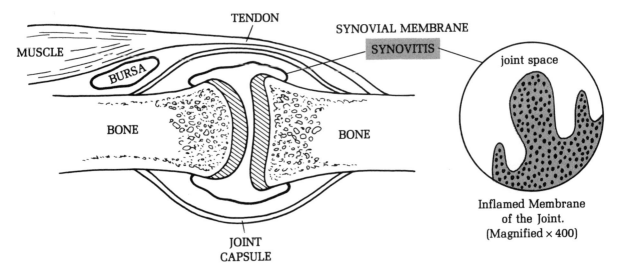

SYNOVITIS

MUSCLE

TENDON

SYNOVIAL MEMBRANE

SYNOVITIS

BURSA

BONE

BONE

JOINT
CAPSULE

joint space

Inflamed Membrane
of the Joint.
(Magnified × 400)

The inflammation of synovitis is located in the lining membrane of the joint, the synovium. This normally thin tissue can become more than one-quarter inch thick, due to the invasion by millions of tiny inflammatory cells. The enzymes released by the inflammation slowly digest the joint parts over many years.

Synovitis is the major problem in rheumatoid arthritis, in juvenile rheumatoid arthritis, in lupus, and in psoriatic arthritis.

Rheumatoid arthritis is more than just arthritis. Indeed, many doctors call it "rheumatoid disease" to emphasize the widespread nature of this process. The name is trying awkwardly to say the same thing; the term *rheum* refers to the stiffness, body aching, and fatigue that often accompany rheumatoid arthritis. Patients with RA often describe feeling much like they have a virus, with fatigue and aching in the muscles, except that, unlike a usual viral illness, the condition may persist for months or even years.

About one-half of one percent of our population has rheumatoid arthritis, some one million individuals in the United States. Most of these people (about three-quarters) are women. The condition usually appears in middle life, in the forties or fifties, although it can begin at any age. Rheumatoid arthritis in children is quite different and is described in the next section. Rheumatoid arthritis has been medically identified for about 200 years, although bone changes in the skeletons of some Mexican Indian groups suggest that the disease may have been around for thousands of years.

Since RA is so common, and because it can sometimes be severe, it is a major national health problem. It can result in difficulties with employment, problems with daily activities, and can severely strain family relationships. In its most severe forms, and without good treatment, it can result in deformities of the joints. Fortunately, most people with RA do well and lead essentially normal lives. Fear of rheumatoid arthritis, sometimes greatly exaggerated, can be as harmful as the disease itself.

Synovitis is the first and truest kind of arthritis, and rheumatoid arthritis is a perfect example of this problem. In RA, the synovial membrane lining the joint becomes inflamed. We don't have a good explanation as to why this inflammation starts, but the cells in the membrane divide and grow and inflammatory cells come into the joint from other parts of the body. Because of the mass of these inflammatory cells, the joint appears swollen and feels puffy or boggy to the touch. The increased blood flow that is a feature of the inflammation makes the joint warm. The cells release enzymes into the joint space and the enzymes cause further irritation and pain. If the process continues for years, the enzymes may gradually digest the cartilage and bone of the joint.

This, then, is synovitis, a process in which inflammation of the joint membrane, over many years, can cause damage to the joint itself.

Features

Swelling and pain in one or more joints, lasting at least six weeks, are first requirements for a diagnosis of rheumatoid arthritis. Usually, both sides of the body are affected similarly and the arthritis is said to be "symmetrical." Often there are slight differences between the two sides, usually the right side being slightly worse in right-handed people and vice versa. Occasionally, the condition skips about in an erratic fashion. The wrists and knuckles are almost always involved, the knees and the joints of the ball of the foot are often involved as well, and any joint can be affected. Of the knuckles, those at the base of the fingers are most frequently painful, while the joints at the ends of the fingers are often spared. Swelling of the middle joints of the fingers often is described as "spindle-shaped" and is sometimes called *fusiform*.

Nodules, usually between the size of a pea and a mothball, may form beneath the skin. These rheumatoid nodules are most commonly located near the elbow at the place where you rest your arms on the table, but they can pop up anywhere. Each represents an inflammation of a small blood vessel. They come and go during the course of the illness and usually are not a big problem. They do tend to occur in people with the most severe kinds of RA. Rarely, they become sore or infected, particularly if they are located around the ankle. Even more rarely, they form in the lungs or elsewhere in the body.

Laboratory tests sometimes can help the doctor recognize rheumatoid arthritis. The *rheumatoid factor* or *latex* (see page 137) is the most commonly used test. Although this test may be negative in the first several months, it is eventually positive in about 80 percent of RA patients. The rheumatoid factor is actually an antibody to certain body proteins and can sometimes be found in patients with other diseases.

The *sed rate* is another frequently used test. This test is called in full an *erythrocyte sedimentation rate* and the name sometimes is abbreviated ESR (p. 136). It doesn't help in diagnosis, but it does help tell how serious the disease is. A high sed rate suggests that the disease is quite active. The joint fluid is sometimes examined in rheumatoid arthritis in order to look at the inflammatory cells or to make sure that the joint is not infected with bacteria.

X-rays (p. 140) can help the doctor determine if damage to the bones or cartilage has occurred. Some doctors like to get baseline X-rays to compare with later X-rays; we prefer to minimize the total number of X-rays. It is unusual for changes to be seen in the bones or cartilage in the first few months of the disease, even when it is most severe.

Most patients with RA notice problems in addition to those of the joints themselves. Usually, these are general problems such as muscle aches, fatigue, muscle stiffness (particularly in the morning), and even a low fever. Morning stiffness is often considered a hallmark of RA, and is sometimes termed the *gel phenomenon*. After a rest period or even after just sitting motionless for a few minutes, the whole body feels stiff and difficult to move. After a period of loosening up, motion becomes easier and less painful. Patients often have problems with fluid accumulation, particularly around the ankles. Occasionally, the rheumatoid disease may attack other body tissues, including the whites of the eyes, the nerves, the small arteries, and the lungs. An anemia (low red blood cell count) is quite common, although it is seldom severe enough to require any treatment.

There can be unusual features due to the synovitis. A *Baker cyst* can form behind the knee and may feel like a tumor. It is just the joint sac full of fluid, but it can extend down into the back of the calf and may cause pain like a blood clot. The carpal-tunnel syndrome (see problem 16 of Part III) involves pressure by the synovitis on a nerve at the wrist. Both of these conditions can occur in patients without rheumatoid arthritis.

Rheumatoid arthritis is one of the most complicated and mysterious diseases known. It is a challenge to patient and physician alike. Fortunately, the course of RA can be dramatically altered in most patients. More so than with any other form of arthritis, if you have RA, you need to develop an effective partnership with your physician to combat its effects.

Prognosis

Rheumatoid arthritis is the condition that most people think of when they hear the word *arthritis*. The image that comes to mind is of a person in a wheelchair, with swollen knees and twisted hands. True, most such patients have rheumatoid arthritis. On balance, rheumatoid arthritis is the most destructive kind of arthritis known. Erosions of the bone itself, rupture of tendons, and slippage of the joints can result in crippling. But most patients with rheumatoid arthritis do very, very much better than this. In fact, only one in six patients with RA develops any crippling or deformities at all. And it is probable that most of these could have been prevented by good, early treatment.

The course of patients with RA usually falls into one of three patterns. The first, and best, is that of a brief illness lasting at most a few months and leaving no disability; this course is sometimes called *monocyclic*. The second involves a series of episodes of illness, separated by periods of being entirely well. This is sometimes termed *polycyclic* and usually does not result in very much physical impairment. The third, termed *chronic*, is a more constant disease lasting a number of years, sometimes for life. Probably the majority of patients with rheumatoid arthritis have this chronic form, but, even here, serious crippling is unusual. Initially it is difficult to be certain which pattern will follow, but a chronic course is suggested by the presence of the rheumatoid factor on a blood test and is strongly suggested if the condition has continued to progress for an entire year.

Often it is hard for patients and relatives to appreciate that even the worst forms of rheumatoid arthritis tend to get better with time. The arthritis tends to become less aggressive. The synovitis is less active and the fatigue and stiffness decrease. New joints are not likely to become involved after several years of the disease. But, even though the disease is less violent, any destruction of bones and ligaments that occurred in earlier years will persist. Thus, deformities do not improve, even though no new damage is occurring. Hence, it is extremely important to treat the disease correctly in the early years, so that the joints will work well after the disease activity subsides.

Treatment

Treatment programs for rheumatoid arthritis are often complicated and can be very confusing. In this section, we broadly outline techniques for sound management. Chapter 12 describes each treatment and provides more details. The combination of measures best for you needs to be worked out with your doctor. It has been said that the person who has himself for a doctor has a fool for a patient. In many areas of medicine, and for some kinds of arthritis, this is not true—you can do just as well looking after yourself. But, with rheumatoid arthritis, you do need a doctor. Indeed, if your rheumatoid arthritis is at all severe, you may want to be seen, at least occasionally, by a specialist in arthritis, a rheumatologist.

First, some common sense. Your rheumatoid arthritis may be with you, on and off, for months or years. The best treatments are those that will help you maintain a life that is as nearly normal as possible. Often the worst treatments are those that offer immediate relief, since they may allow joint damage to go on or may cause delayed side effects that ultimately make you feel worse. So, you must develop some patience with the disease and with its management. You have to adjust your thinking to operate in the same slow time frame that the disease uses. You and your doctor will want to be anticipating problems before they occur, so that they may be avoided. The adjustment to a long-term illness, with the necessity to plan treatment programs that may take months to get results, is a difficult psychological task. It is easy to understand in principle, but very difficult to put into daily action. This adjustment will be one of your hardest jobs in battling your arthritis.

Synovitis is the underlying problem. Inflammation of the joint membrane releases enzymes that very slowly damage the joint structures. Good treatment reduces this inflammation and stops the damage. Painkillers can increase comfort but do not decrease the arthritis. In fact, pain per se helps to protect the joints by discouraging too much use. So, in RA, it is important to treat pain by treating the inflammation that causes the pain. By and large, analgesics such as codeine, Percodan, Darvon, Talwin, or Demerol must be avoided.

The proper balance between rest and exercise is an essential part of treatment. Rest reduces the inflammation, and this is good. But rest also lets joints get stiff and muscles get weak. With too much rest, tendons become less strong and bones get softer. Obviously, this is bad. So, moderation is the basic principle. It may help you to know that your body usually gives you the right signals about what to do and what not to do. If it hurts too much, don't do it. If you don't seem to have much problem with an activity, go ahead.

A particularly painful joint may require a splint to help it rest. Still, you will want to exercise the joint by moving it gently in different directions to prevent it from getting stiff and you will not want to use a splint for too long—you may decide to use it just at night. As the joint gets better, begin using the joint, gently at first but slowly progressing to more and more activity. In general, favor activities that build good muscle tone, not those that build great muscle strength. Walking and swimming are better than furniture moving and weight lifting, since tasks requiring a lot of strength put a lot of stress across the joint. And regular exercises done daily are better than occasional sprees of activity that unduly stress joints not ready for so much exertion.

Common sense and a regular, long-term program are the keys to success. Should you take a nap after lunch? Yes, if you're tired. Should you undertake some particular outing? Go on a trip? You know your regular daily activity level. Common sense will answer most such questions. Full normal activity should be approached gradually with a long-term conditioning program that includes rest when needed and graded increases in activity during nonresting periods.

Physical therapists and occupational therapists can often help with specific advice and helpful hints. The best therapists will help you develop your own program for home exercise and will teach you the exercises and activities that will help your joints. However, don't expect the therapist to do your program for you. Your rest and exercise program cannot consist solely of formal sessions at a rehabilitation facility. You must take the responsibility to build the habits that will, on a daily basis, protect and strengthen your joints.

Medications are required by most patients with rheumatoid arthritis and often must be continued for months or years. By and large, the most powerful drugs have the worst side effects. So, most good physicians begin with the simplest and the safest drugs and use more hazardous drugs only if the simpler measures are not sufficient. Most patients will not require the more powerful drugs.

Aspirin is the most valuable single drug, when used correctly. Its use is described in detail in Chapter 12, and every patient with RA should become very familiar with the uses of aspirin. Aspirin, used correctly (p. 98), is a strong anti-inflammatory drug with an acceptable level of side effects. Drugs roughly similar to aspirin are called *nonsteroidal anti-inflammatory drugs* and are also frequently used. Examples of such drugs are Motrin (p. 102), Nalfon (p. 103), Tolectin (p. 104), Naprosyn (p. 104), and Indocin (p. 102).

Antimalarial drugs such as chloroquine or Plaquenil (p. 111) are sometimes used next, if the anti-inflammatory agents have not been enough. Gold injections (p. 113) are often helpful if the previous drugs have not been sufficient and sometimes result in complete disappearance of the arthritis. Penicillamine (p. 114) is an experimental drug that also can result in dramatic improvement.

Corticosteroids, most frequently prednisone (p. 108), are strong hormones with formidable long-term side effects. Their use is controversial in rheumatoid arthritis; some physicians feel that they should almost never be used and others use them only in very small doses. Immunosuppressant drugs, such as Cytoxan (p. 124), Imuran (p. 125), or chlorambucil (p. 124), are powerful, experimental, and hazardous; some physicians think that these drugs are too dangerous to use in rheumatoid arthritis, and all agree that they should be used with caution. Steroids and immunosuppressants are sometimes needed for severe systemic complications, such as nerve damage or eye damage.

Surgery sometimes can restore the function of a damaged joint. Hip replacement, knee replacement, synovectomy of the knee, metatarsal head resection, and synovectomy of the knuckles are among the most frequent operations; these are discussed in Chapter 13.

If you have rheumatoid arthritis, proceed now to Part II, "Managing Your Arthritis," page 87.

ARTHRITIS IN CHILDREN (JUVENILE ARTHRITIS, JRA)

Children get arthritis too. In fact, over 100,000 children in the United States have an important kind of arthritis called juvenile rheumatoid arthritis (JRA). This name, however, is misleading, since it suggests that these children have a disease similar to rheumatoid arthritis in adults. For the most part, these children have a quite different set of problems and require quite different treatment; the outlook for their complete recovery is better than that for persons with adult rheumatoid arthritis.

Children, of course, lead very active lives and continually do things to their joints, muscles, and back. They fall down, sprain their ankles, and experience a variety of temporary aches and pains; these are not really arthritis. Occasionally a child will be born with an abnormality in a knee, hip, or elsewhere. Again, this is not really arthritis. Very rarely, a child will have a joint infected with bacteria (most commonly the staphylococcus) which causes a severe infectious arthritis like that discussed later (p. 48). An adolescent will sometimes develop arthritis due to infection with the gonococcal bacteria. These problems are true arthritis, but they are acute forms. They develop rapidly and last less than six weeks in their entirety. In this section, we are concerned with arthritis of longer duration in children.

Three forms of juvenile arthritis are now generally recognized. The first is an arthritis that occurs in only one joint or, at most, in two, three, or four. The second is an illness that is more impressive for its high fever and its skin rash than for the arthritis itself. The third is an arthritis involving many joints and resembling the rheumatoid arthritis seen in adults.

Beyond these major subtypes, there are other kinds of chronic arthritis in children. Acute rheumatic fever is a completely different disease that must not be confused with other forms of childhood arthritis. And some kinds of attachment arthritis described in Chapter 3, such as ankylosing spondylitis, can occur in children.

Features

The following paragraphs describe the features of the three types of juvenile arthritis, as well as of acute rheumatic fever.

Monoarticular arthritis simply means arthritis that involves only one joint. Most frequently, this joint is a knee. *Pauciarticular* or *oligoarticular* are similar words that mean "few joints" and allow for the fact that this type of arthritis may involve one, two, three, or even four joints. Usually the joints involved are large ones. Most children with pauciarticular arthritis feel generally well, except for their swollen, sore, affected joints. In a few instances, there may be involvement of the eye. Many doctors will ask an ophthalmologist to perform periodically a *slit lamp* examination of the eye to detect any eye problems. In this procedure, a thin beam of light is projected obliquely onto the eye through a narrow slit to permit examination of the eye by a magnifying lens.

The *systemic* form of juvenile arthritis is far more dramatic. This form has been called *Still's disease.* A child may suddenly develop very high fever, as high as 106°F, and may be very ill with fatigue, muscle aching, and perhaps a fine, red skin rash. The liver, spleen, and lymph nodes may be enlarged and the disease may involve other organs as well. There may be just a little arthritis, quite a bit of arthritis, or no arthritis at all. The attack may last days or weeks and disappear as quickly and mysteriously as it came. A few months or years later it may recur again, and again, and again. Eventually there are always attacks of arthritis along with the episodes, but these may not appear for several years.

Polyarticular juvenile arthritis affects many joints and usually comes on slowly in children approaching adolescence. The arthritis is usually experienced equally on both sides of the body and frequently affects the wrists and knuckles as well as the knees and other joints. This form is characterized by intense inflammation of the joint membrane and synovitis, and closely resembles the rheumatoid arthritis seen in adults.

Acute rheumatic fever follows a streptococcal infection, usually a "strep throat." It is a less frequent illness now than it was a few years ago. The possibility of acute rheumatic fever is the major reason that throat cultures are taken and that penicillin is sometimes given to treat sore throats, since rheumatic fever can be prevented by such treatment. Acute rheumatic fever is an allergic (immunologic) reaction of the body against the strep bacteria infection that occurred several weeks before the rheumatic fever. Antibodies attack the joints (and sometimes the heart valves and other parts of the body).

This arthritis is termed *migratory* in that it will, for example, appear in one joint, such as the knee, then migrate to a shoulder, then to a wrist, and then to the other knee. Affected children may have a heart murmur, a fever, or an unusual red skin rash with sharp, irregular borders.

Laboratory tests for juvenile arthritis are not very helpful. By and large, all of the usual tests for arthritis are negative. Even in children with the polyarticular arthritis most closely resembling adult rheumatoid arthritis, only a minority have a positive rheumatoid-factor test. The sedimentation rate (p. 136) is often elevated, but this indicates the severity of the inflammation and not the accuracy of the diagnosis. With acute rheumatic fever, a blood test can confirm that a streptococcal infection has occurred recently.

Similarly, X-rays are usually not very helpful. This is a fortunate thing, since we do not like to X-ray children unnecessarily. Destruction of the joints sufficient to cause X-ray changes to the bone is uncommon in children. Watching the course of the disease with time often provides the most important diagnostic clues. Does the arthritis stay in the original joints? Are there associated skin rashes or fever? Does the arthritis come in recurring attacks? Does it tend to involve both sides of the body equally? Such questions require patience on the part of parent, child, and physician. The patience is usually rewarded by a good outcome for the child.

Prognosis

Many of us have the idea that arthritis, once encountered, is present for life. This is not true. When a child develops arthritis, the concern of parents, child, and even the child's school is naturally intense. Fortunately, reassurance can be strong. In children, the disease usually disappears entirely with time. Most children with juvenile arthritis will grow into normal adults without any leftover bone or joint problems. This does not mean that parent or child can relax. Hard work is required to prevent development of permanent stiffness, particularly when a period of active arthritis coincides with one of rapid growth. The long-term outlook, however, is good.

This is particularly true of the first two categories of juvenile arthritis. At least two-thirds of children with monoarticular or pauciarticular disease will have no problems with arthritis as adults. Even with the dramatic systemic form (Still's disease) a similar two-thirds of children will have no problems as adults. The outlook is not quite as favorable for children with polyarticular arthritis—about half of these children will continue to require treatment for arthritis in adult life.

Acute rheumatic fever does not cause joint destruction and arthritis continuing into adult life is extremely unlikely.

Treatment

Drug treatment of arthritis in children centers around the considered use of aspirin (p. 98). Aspirin, in anti-inflammatory doses, will satisfactorily control the arthritis in the great majority of patients, without the potentially severe side effects of other medications. Some of the new anti-inflammatory agents are not yet approved for use in children, and their effects on growth and development are not fully understood.

On the other hand, the effects of the corticosteroids (p. 106) on growth are understood only too well; these agents cause bone growth to stop and can lead to failure to reach adult height. The other well-known side effects of steroids also occur; thus, these drugs must be used only with extreme caution in growing children. Their most justifiable use is in short courses of treatment for the dramatic but brief episodes of illness with Still's disease, or for severe eye problems.

Occasionally, antimalarial compounds (p. 110) or a series of injections of gold salts (p. 113) may be used in treatment of juvenile arthritis. The careful physician, however, relies on aspirin as the major drug for the majority of patients.

Physical therapy and exercise programs, particularly swimming, are very helpful in maintaining muscle tone and mobility in the child with arthritis. Sometimes special arrangements with the child's school are required so that the child doesn't fall behind during the period of time the arthritis is expected to remain active. Since the overall outlook is good, a reasonable plan of management includes attention to keeping the child up with his or her peers, so that when the arthritis subsides, a normal development pattern can be resumed. For many patients, body contact sports and activities (such as basketball) which require a lot of jumping, should be discouraged while the disease is active.

Surgery is seldom required and follows indications similar to those in adults. It is needed only infrequently, because the destructive aspects of the arthritis are less in children. A surgical procedure sometimes required is the removal of the synovium (joint membrane) of the knee, but this is now less frequently performed than a few years ago. "Soft tissue release" procedures to increase motion (capsulotomy) are fairly frequently performed.

Rather rarely, removal of joint fluid through a needle provides some relief. Even more rarely, injection of a corticosteroid preparation into a knee joint or other joint is helpful. Since too many treatments of this kind can accelerate bone destruction, they must be used with caution.

If childhood arthritis is the problem, proceed now to Part II, page 87.

LUPUS (SYSTEMIC LUPUS ERYTHEMATOSUS, SLE)

The word *lupus* means "wolf." The disease is so named because some lupus patients develop a red rash across the nose and cheeks that causes the face to look a little bit like that of a wolf. The full name of the disease, systemic lupus erythematosus, is a bit hard to remember. The *systemic* part refers to the many parts of the body that may be involved by this condition. The term *erythema* refers to the red color of the rash. There is a skin condition with a somewhat similar rash called discoid lupus erythematosus; thus, the word *systemic* serves to emphasize that SLE is a more widespread disease.

Lupus is not always thought of as a form of arthritis. Lupus is described as a "connective-tissue" disease or a "collagen" disease or a "collagen vascular" disease. These terms describe a family of diseases discussed further starting on page 82. About half of lupus patients have arthritis.

Lupus is also considered an *autoimmune* disease—that is, most of the problems seem to come from antibodies created by the body attacking other parts of the body. In the case of the arthritis, it seems as though the body is using its defense systems against outside viruses to attack the lining of its own joints.

This is a highly variable disease. Some patients with lupus aren't even aware of it and require no treatment. Others have a major illness. Lupus has developed a much worse reputation than it deserves, since newspaper, magazine, and television depictions of the disease focus on those few patients with dramatic symptoms rather than on the many who do extremely well without major difficulties.

Features

The arthritis of lupus is a synovitis; it involves inflammation of the lining membrane of the joint. Compared with rheumatoid arthritis, however, the synovitis in less severe. Whereas the patient with rheumatoid arthritis usually has visibly swollen joints that feel spongy to the touch, the joints of a patient with lupus arthritis may appear entirely normal. When we look at the synovial membrane under the microscope, we see that the thick *pannus* (covering membrane) of inflammatory tissue so characteristic of rheumatoid arthritis is not present. Rather, there is a less violent inflammation of the joint membrane. This difference in intensity of the inflammatory response is one reason why the arthritis of lupus is usually not as severe as rheumatoid arthritis.

The joints affected by lupus are almost exactly the same ones affected by rheumatoid arthritis. The wrists, the knuckles at the base of the fingers, and the knuckles in the middle of the fingers are most frequently involved in the upper extremity. In the lower extremity, the knees are most commonly involved. Sometimes the hips may be attacked and, on occasion, there is a problem with the blood supply to the hip joint, causing a complication called *aseptic necrosis.* Although these are the major joints, any other joint in the body may also be involved. The spine is usually spared.

The usual symptom is pain. The joints will be tender when squeezed and sore when moved. As noted, they may not look abnormal at all. The doctor may initially be skeptical about the presence of arthritis, but laboratory tests will help confirm the existence of the disease.

X-rays of the arthritis of lupus are usually normal. In rheumatoid arthritis, the inflammatory process actually erodes the bones, causing little holes to develop near the ends of the bones. With lupus these erosions are very rare, and it is unusual for the arthritis to damage the joint very much.

Lupus is a multisystem disease characterized by autoantibodies. We are currently following about 270 patients with lupus and each has had evidence of abnormal autoantibodies. Additionally, each has had disease of at least two organs out of the seven listed below. Most of these problems are mild or last only a short period.

The *skin* may be affected with rashes or sores. Sometimes there is Raynaud's phenomenon, in which the fingers become blue and white after exposure to cold. Small ulcers may develop inside the mouth. The skin rash may take a characteristic butterfly appearance over the cheeks and it may become worse after exposure to sunlight.

The *joint* disease of lupus was previously discussed. It is a synovitis, but a less violent one than that seen in rheumatoid arthritis. It is unusual to have joint deformity.

The *blood* elements may be affected by the autoantibodies of lupus. The white cells are frequently decreased, a condition termed *leukopenia*. The red cells may be depressed (*anemia*) by an antibody reaction or just by the general effects of the disease. The platelets may be severely depressed (*thrombocytopenia*), leading to bleeding.

The pleura that surrounds the lungs, the pericardium that surrounds the heart, and the peritoneum that surrounds the abdominal cavity are called *serous membranes*. Each of these may be inflamed at times in lupus, the pleura being the most commonly affected (pleurisy).

The *lungs* may, rather rarely, be involved in lupus. This problem resembles a mild pneumonia, but is not caused by germs and clears with anti-inflammatory drugs and without antibiotics.

The *kidneys* pose the major problem with lupus and at least half of patients with lupus have some kidney difficulty. Lupus causes *nephritis* when the autoantibodies form *immune complexes* which collect inside the kidneys.

The *central nervous system* is involved every so often in lupus. Seizures or other nervous or emotional problems may result.

Because lupus is an *immunological* disease, the diagnosis can be assisted by the finding of antibodies in the blood. The most common blood test detects *antinuclear antibodies* which are found in some other diseases but are most characteristic of lupus. This blood test is positive in almost everyone with lupus. Sometimes the sedimentation rate will be elevated, there may be a low white blood count, and many other blood tests may be abnormal.

Prognosis

The arthritis of lupus has a good prognosis. Doctors usually talk about it as being "nondeforming," meaning that injury to the bone is rare and that patients usually do well over a long period of time without any crippling. On the other hand, the arthritis does tend to be persistent and may remain active for many months or years. Ultimately, the activity of the disease begins to subside, but this may require five, ten, or even fifteen years.

Actually, a few patients with lupus arthritis do develop some deformity of the joints, particularly of the hands. These deformities are somewhat different from those of rheumatoid arthritis, because they result from slippage or *subluxation* of the joints rather than destruction. The tendons and ligaments around the joint get a little loose and a certain degree of deformity may result. For example, the fingers may bend backward more than they should, or a finger may be bent backward at the middle knuckle and forward at the last knuckle, giving the appearance of a "swan neck." Usually, the hand will work well even if this problem occurs; serious disability resulting from the arthritis is unusual.

Only a small fraction of all of the things that can possibly happen in lupus will happen to any one person. Patients frequently worry unrealistically about what might next go wrong. The prognosis in lupus has improved now, so that death from the disease is quite unusual. More than 90 percent of all patients with lupus live at least ten years, and the majority live normal life spans. The prognosis depends on the particular kind of lupus. Patients who have the arthritis of lupus or who have the Raynaud's phenomenon (color changes in the hands after exposure to cold) do somewhat better than the average lupus patient, while those who have involvement of the kidneys or central nervous system do a bit worse. But the outlook is now good for all.

Treatment

Treatment of lupus is complicated, since the disease varies considerably from one person to another. Powerful and dangerous drugs such as corticosteroids (p. 106) and immunosuppressants (p. 123) are required for some patients with SLE. However, usually the disease can be managed with either low doses of corticosteroids, the anti-inflammatory agents discussed later, aspirin (p. 98), hydroxychloroquine (p. 111), or other reasonably safe drugs. Perhaps a quarter of lupus patients require little treatment and may do better without even these mild drugs.

Life-style, as in all of the rheumatic diseases, can make a significant difference in the effectiveness of a treatment program. Worry can become as serious a malady as the disease itself. While certainty about prognosis is not always possible, the odds are good for every patient and minimum disruption in life-style is the goal.

The tendency in past years to counsel strict avoidance of the sun and strict avoidance of overactivity has now been greatly relaxed. We urge patients to stay out of the sun only if being out in the sun causes a flare-up of their disease, and rest only if they are tired. We have been rewarded with many patients living confident, productive lives who, in more restrictive years, would have been socially quarantined.

Knowledge that the arthritis is unlikely to result in crippling and that the great majority of patients can lead essentially normal lives is very helpful to many patients. A good long-term relationship with a physician familiar with this disease is important. The physician will want to follow the patient to ensure that complicating disease of other body organs does not occur.

Surgery is seldom required. Occasionally, operations to realign the tendons of the finger joints are performed. And, if aseptic necrosis of the hip has developed, surgery for the hip joint, usually total replacement of the hip, is sometimes required.

If you have lupus, proceed now to Part II, page 87.

PSORIATIC ARTHRITIS

Psoriasis is a skin condition well known to most people because it is so common. Red, scaling patches, which sometimes bleed when injured, are common near the elbows and knees, but can occur any place in the body. Often the fingernails or an area around the fingernails are affected with these psoriatic skin patches. In cases of extensive psoriasis, much of the body may be covered with the skin lesions. In psoriasis, the lower layers of the skin contain cells that divide more rapidly than normal, causing patches of thicker skin to grow and then scale off from the top.

It is not as well known that arthritis can occur with psoriasis. Probably some 10 percent of patients with psoriasis also have some arthritis. Arthritis experts have argued for years about the exact forms of arthritis that can accompany psoriasis and the picture is not yet totally clear. Nevertheless, at this time there is nearly unanimous agreement that particular types of arthritis are directly related to the skin condition.

Part of the confusion has been generated by the fact that both psoriasis and several forms of arthritis are quite common. Hence, just as a matter of coincidence, you would expect to see some people with both psoriasis and arthritis. This will of course be most common with the most frequently occurring forms of arthritis: ankylosing spondylitis, rheumatoid arthritis, gout, and osteoarthritis. Since these coincidences do occur, it is possible to have psoriasis and arthritis without having psoriatic arthritis. If your arthritis more closely resembles one of these other types, it may have nothing to do with the psoriasis condition.

Features

Psoriatic arthritis is part synovitis and part attachment arthritis, so it is discussed immediately preceding the next chapter on attachment arthritis.

In comparison with rheumatoid arthritis, psoriatic arthritis is usually not the same on both sides of the body and it affects different sets of joints. Whereas rheumatoid arthritis affects the middle knuckles more frequently, psoriatic arthritis attacks the end joints of the fingers. The joints involved by psoriatic arthritis are frequently spotty and irregular in their distribution. For example, the second finger of one hand and the third finger and thumb of the other may be affected.

Rheumatoid arthritis frequently results in overall tiredness and fatigue, with pronounced stiffness in the morning and with wasting of the calcium in the bones. In psoriatic arthritis these features are less common. The patient with psoriatic arthritis frequently feels perfectly well, except for the problems with the skin and joints, and not excessively fatigued. Further, bone strength usually is preserved throughout the course of the disease.

Some patients with psoriatic arthritis will experience an unusual feature of the disease termed a *sausage digit*. This is a finger or a toe swollen uniformly from beginning to end, so that it resembles a sausage. It may be twice the size of an adjacent finger or toe. This results from synovitis of the joints of the digit together with swelling of the soft tissues between the joints. The sausage digit occurs only in psoriatic arthritis and in the condition called Reiter's syndrome discussed in the next section.

Pain in the heel or low back pain sometimes accompanies psoriatic arthritis, although these problems are unusual in rheumatoid arthritis. In some patients, the joint problems will come and go as the skin problem improves or gets worse; this relationship is not constant.

There are no good laboratory tests for psoriatic arthritis. The skin disease is usually easily identified by examination, but can be confirmed by looking at a biopsy of skin under the microscope. Blood tests for rheumatoid factor (*latex fixation*) are negative. The sedimentation rate may be elevated or not.

X-rays may show bone erosions similar to those of rheumatoid arthritis. More characteristic, however, is the formation of new bone along the sides of existing bones, giving a fluffy X-ray appearance. Erosions sometimes result in "whittling" of the ends of the bones, so that a bone end which should be approximately square develops a point almost like a pencil. X-rays of the back may show changes similar to ankylosing spondylitis in the sacroiliac joints and in the spine. However, involvement of the sacroiliac joints is often spotty; only one side may be involved or the two sides may be involved but with different degrees of severity. When involvement of the spine occurs, just one side of a particular vertebra may be affected.

Prognosis

Throughout this book there is an emphasis on the variability in prognosis for arthritis. It is important to realize that very few patients are severely crippled by arthritis. Psoriatic arthritis easily wins the distinction of being the most variable of all of the rheumatic diseases. In the great majority of patients the disease is mild; it might even be termed trivial. Medication may be required at some times and there may be some stiffness in one or another joint. But the arthritis is not as severe a problem as is the skin.

On the other hand, in the very worst cases, a condition that is probably the most crippling arthritis of all occurs. This condition, called rather bizarrely *arthritis mutilans*, affects less than one-tenth of one percent of all patients with psoriasis and arthritis. It is thus a very rare happening and should not pose a major worry for the most patients. Some such patients have a combination of the worst possibilities of rheumatoid arthritis and ankylosing spondylitis. We believe that most such cases can now be prevented by correct early treatment.

Because fatigue, tiredness, and stiffness are much less prominent in psoriatic arthritis than in rheumatoid arthritis, almost all patients are able to work and play normally throughout their illness. Relatively few will have difficulty with employment, with homemaking, or with most of their other daily activities.

Patients should maintain a schedule of essentially normal activities unless a particular problem mandates some limitation. Techniques of protecting involved joints are important, as is exercising these joints through their entire range of motion to prevent stiffening. Rest of the entire body, sometimes important in rheumatoid arthritis, is seldom needed, and fatigue is usually not present. Beyond this, the same general treatment principles apply as for rheumatoid arthritis.

Drug treatment for psoriatic arthritis has a slightly different spectrum than that of rheumatoid arthritis. Indomethacin (p. 102), phenylbutazone (p. 101), and other anti-inflammatory agents frequently are better than aspirin in this condition, although the reverse is often true in rheumatoid arthritis. Aspirin (p. 98) is not as consistent a treatment with the arthritis of psoriasis. Corticosteroids (p. 106), such as prednisone, are not frequently useful in psoriatic arthritis. Although they may temporarily improve the skin condition, it sometimes becomes worse on discontinuation of the steroid; most doctors try to avoid these drugs whenever possible. Controversy reigns concerning the use of gold shots (p. 113), with some physicians of the opinion that increase in the skin disease may be caused by gold injections while others use these injections frequently and apparently safely.

For severe cases, the immunosuppressant drugs, even though experimental, have shown considerable promise. In psoriatic arthritis they have the advantage of being effective against both the skin and the joint problems. Since psoriatic arthritis patients are constitutionally strong, these powerful drugs are usually well tolerated with few side effects. Methotrexate (p. 125) and azathioprine (p. 125) are most frequently used; their use should be reserved for the most severe cases, with full and frank discussion about the potential side effects between patient and physician.

Finally, one may treat psoriatic arthritis by treating the psoriasis. Since in some patients there is a linkage between the state of the skin disease and the state of the arthritis, aggressive treatment efforts using appropriate tars, creams, drugs, and ultraviolet light are sometimes successful in reducing the level of activity of the arthritis.

If your problem is psoriatic arthritis, proceed now to Part II, page 87.

Attachment Arthritis:

Inflammation of the Joint Attachments

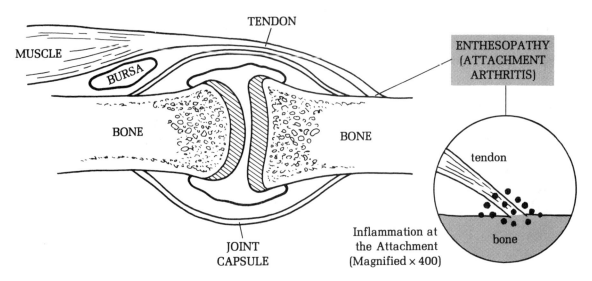

ATTACHMENT ARTHRITIS

The inflammation of an "enthesopathy" is located where a ligament or a tendon attaches to the bone. The small dark inflammatory cells invade this area and cause pain and tissue damage. For this book, we introduce the term "attachment arthritis" to explain this process.

Ankylosing spondylitis, Reiter's Disease, and sometimes psoriatic arthritis or arthritis associated with bowel disease are forms of attachment arthritis. These diseases are related to a particular gene and run in families.

ANKYLOSING SPONDYLITIS

Ankylosing spondylitis has a jawbreaker of a name. This disease has gone by a variety of other names during the 3,000 years that it is known to have existed as a human disease. In this century, it was called Marie-Strumpel disease, after the two doctors who first described the condition fully. Later it became known as rheumatoid spondylitis. Since this name suggested that it was related to rheumatoid arthritis, which it is not, the name has been changed to ankylosing spondylitis, or AS for short.

A "poker spine" is the feature that most people remember about this disease. Severely affected patients have a very stiff back, like a poker, and are unable to bend. Unlike rheumatoid arthritis, which affects the joints of the hands and feet, ankylosing spondylitis affects the central parts of the body. More importantly, the disease is distinguished from rheumatoid arthritis by being an *enthesopathy* instead of a synovitis.

I am using the term *attachment arthritis* in place of *enthesopathy* simply because it is easier to remember. Remember that the inflammation is not in the lining membrane of the joint but rather where the ligaments and tendons attach to the bone. Thus, the inflammation is not *in* the joint but is right *next to* the joint. Understanding this difference will make clear why spondylitis affects certain parts of the body, why it causes stiffness more than pain, and why it responds to different medicines than those used for rheumatoid arthritis. "Attachment arthritis" is a new term made up for this book to help you understand the process better; your doctor will be familiar with the process but possibly not with the new term.

Ankylosing spondylitis is a genetic disease. The gene region that predisposes to ankylosing spondylitis has been identified. This disease tends to occur in families; over one-half of patients with ankylosing spondylitis have another family member with the disease. The gene region associated with the disease is called *B27*. If you have the gene, our data suggests that you may have as high as a 20 percent chance of developing ankylosing spondylitis at some time during your life. If you don't have the gene, for all practical purposes you are immune to ankylosing spondylitis. Nearly 100 percent of white patients with ankylosing spondylitis have this gene, the proportion is lower in Blacks, some Indian tribes, and some other races.

About seven percent of white individuals in the United States carry the B27 gene region. Thus, ankylosing spondylitis is a common disease that may occur in more than one percent of the population of the United States. Genetic factors are often closely associated with race, and B27 is no exception. Some Indian tribes have as much as 50 percent frequency of the gene, while B27 is very rare in the black race. As expected, these Indian tribes have a very high frequency of spondylitis, while the disease almost never affects black individuals.

Identification of the gene region is allowing research on this disease to proceed at a rapid pace. It seems likely that the cause of this form of arthritis will be known within a few years, permitting even more effective treatment.

Features

Not all of the joints of the body have a synovial lining. Some consist simply of fibers that bridge across the joint and allow limited movement. Since ankylosing spondylitis is an attachment arthritis, it affects such joints more than those with the synovial lining. The sacroiliac (SI) joint attaches the sacrum at the bottom of the spine to the pelvic bones by means of many strong fibers. Thus, it is not surprising that the sacroiliac joints are the most involved joints in ankylosing spondylitis. Sacroiliitis is the hallmark of this disease, and almost all patients have sacroiliac-caused back pain. The pain usually has a component of stiffness and the stiffness is worse in the morning. The disease comes on slowly, usually beginning around age 20. Usually, the back pain is not associated with any accident or injury.

Over time, the condition tends to move from the lower regions of the spine toward the higher. It may involve the fibrous joints that attach the ribs to the spine and the ribs to the breastbone. It may reach to the neck. If it extends to the joints of the limbs, usually just the hips or perhaps the shoulders are involved. In severe cases, the attachment of the skull to the neck can be ankylosed and frozen.

The inflammation at the ends of the ligaments results in stiffness, and it hurts to move. After a period of stiffness and pain, a bony bridge grows between the parts and the area becomes totally rigid. Obviously, this fusion stops motion, but it has the beneficial effect of removing pain; pain is experienced only in areas that are still able to move. Rheumatoid arthritis can cause destruction of the bones around a joint, whereas ankylosing spondylitis fuses the intact bones together.

The most important diagnostic test for AS is an X-ray of the sacroiliac joints (p. 141). Usually the disease, if it has been present for two or more years, can be conclusively diagnosed by a single X-ray of the pelvis with particular attention paid to the state of the sacroiliac joints.

When the doctor is examining the patient, stiffness in the back may be measured by tests of back flexion. The chest may not expand as fully as it should, because of involvement of the joints at the ends of the ribs. This can be detected by putting a tape measure around the chest at the level of the nipples and noting the difference between the chest circumference after the biggest possible intake of breath and after blowing all of the air out of the chest. Normally the chest circumference changes by at least two inches, but many patients with ankylosing spondylitis will have a change of less than one-half inch. Such simple tests can strongly suggest a diagnosis of AS, but X-rays are required to confirm it.

In contrast, other tests are not as helpful. Basically, almost all laboratory tests are normal. The sedimentation rate is elevated in some patients but is normal in others. The B27 test for the underlying gene (p. 138) will be positive in almost everyone. The problem with this test is that, since the gene is found in seven percent of the white population, a positive test for the gene does not necessarily prove ankylosing spondylitis. Most people with the B27 gene are well.

In a few patients, particularly those who are most severely affected, ankylosing spondylitis will cause an inflammation of the eye with redness and pain, may result in damage to the aortic valve of the heart, or may be associated with cavities in the lungs. In severely affected patients, when the rib cage does not move well, pneumonia may develop.

The bony fusion can be extensive in the most severely affected patients and can lead to the creation of a single giant bone that includes the pelvis, the spine, the skull, and the ribs, without any motion at all in the central part of the body. The fusion is usually symmetrical, with both sacroiliac joints involved to the same extent and with both sides of the spine and rib cage equally involved.

Prognosis

Ankylosing spondylitis is most frequently a mild condition and is not considered a serious problem by either patient or physician. For example, the diagnosis is often not made until around age 40, while the disease began some 20 years earlier. Some studies suggest that there are ten times as many patients with ankylosing spondylitis who are undiagnosed in the United States as there are patients who have been diagnosed. Early studies that suggested the disease is found almost entirely in men have come under some attack; it is now felt that the disease may be nearly as common in women, although in a milder form.

Almost all patients with ankylosing spondylitis lead vigorous, physically active lives without major limitation from the disease. Patients with spondylitis usually have normal employment records without undue absences. The degree to which fusion of the back is consistent with a normal life-style is amazing. Patients with ankylosing spondylitis usually adapt very well to the presence of a chronic disease and do not experience major difficulties from it.

Probably fewer than one out of one hundred patients with spondylitis progresses to serious limitation or deformity. Death due to the disease is very unusual and almost all patients have a normal life span. Death can occasionally occur from a severe problem with the aortic valve or from a serious infection of the lungs, but only in those few patients who have the most severe forms of the disease.

The most common significant limitation is a fusion of the neck in a flexed position, limiting the person's ability to raise the head. The hips are involved in a few percent of patients, and if this involvement is serious, some limitation of mobility may result.

Treatment

The approach to treatment follows logically from the discussion above. Since the disease is working to fuse parts of the body together, the therapeutic response involves stretching those body parts. Motion exercises with stretching in all directions should be performed several times daily. Many physicians recommend deep-breathing exercises in order to slow the fusion of the rib joints. Posture is as important as exercise. Patients should sleep on their back without a pillow, so that the spine is rested in the most useful position; even if fusion occurs, it will happen in the position of best function. Good chairs and other commonsense measures are important. I have seen patients who could sleep only on one side and who used several pillows develop a neck deformity with the head cocked to one side. Clearly, this could have been avoided. Anticipating the possibility that the motion of the chest might be limited at some point, we urge patients to stop cigarette smoking, since smoking can damage the lungs and aggravate the later tendency to develop lung infections.

Since this is a genetic disease, many patients ask about the risk to other family members or about the advisability of having children. While these decisions must be made by the individual, medical advice is reassuring. If an individual with ankylosing spondylitis is married to an individual who is negative for the B27 gene, then any particular child has a one in ten chance of developing the disease, and a one in two chance of carrying the gene. Of family members who may be affected, most will have mild and almost undetectable disease. Since the gene appears to cause no other form of illness and since patients with ankylosing spondylitis are frequently noteworthy for their good general health, there seems little reason to counsel patients not to have a family.

The symptoms of ankylosing spondylitis can be strikingly decreased by medical treatment and patients with ankylosing spondylitis should be under medical treatment as long as they are experiencing pain or stiffness. Indomethacin (p. 102) and phenylbutazone (p. 101) are among the more useful drugs. Aspirin (p. 98) does not seem to be as helpful in ankylosing spondylitis as it is in rheumatoid arthritis, and it is used less frequently. Some of the new anti-inflammatory agents (p. 100) appear to be helpful on occasion. Corticosteroids probably should never be used for this disease.

There is medical controversy as to whether these drugs actually prevent the fusion of bones. The drugs relieve symptoms in most patients at any stage of the disease. Over the short term—weeks or months—they clearly improve the motion of the spine and allow the patient to exercise to a wider range of motion. No adequate studies of the long-term effects of these drugs have been performed, but reports suggest that patients who have had regular medical treatment end up with less stiffness than those who have not. The control of symptoms allows greater degrees of motion.

If you have ankylosing spondylitis, proceed now to Part II, page 87.

REITER'S SYNDROME

A German army physician, Hans Reiter, first described this syndrome during World War I. Reiter described a disease with three features—an arthritis, a painful inflammation (*conjunctivitis*) of the eye, and a discharge from the penis (*urethritis*)—in an army lieutenant. Later observers added a fourth feature sometimes characteristic of the disease, a particular skin rash called *keratoderma blennorrhagica.* Reiter's syndrome is relatively rare compared to most of the forms of arthritis described in this book, but is the second most common cause of arthritis in young men in their late teens or twenties. (Ankylosing spondylitis is first.)

The same gene (B27) that is almost always present in ankylosing spondylitis is nearly always present in Reiter's syndrome (p. 38). Reiter's patients have this gene from 70 percent to 90 percent of the time, compared with 7 percent in the white population. Like ankylosing spondylitis, Reiter's syndrome is unusual in the black race. Occasionally, family members may have the disease, underscoring the genetic effect, but family members are more likely to have ankylosing spondylitis than the rarer Reiter's syndrome.

Infection seems to cause Reiter's syndrome. The infection may occur several weeks before the development of the arthritis, the urethritis, and the conjunctivitis, and the infections seem to fall into two broad categories. In the United States, there is usually a sexual exposure to the disease shortly before the development of discharge from the penis, which is usually the first symptom. Reiter's syndrome is not considered a definite venereal disease, but most physicians think venereal exposure to be a likely cause. The infection appears to cause Reiter's syndrome in those susceptible individuals with the B27 gene.

The second form follows episodes of diarrhea. This form can occur in epidemics and is most frequently related to *Shigella dysentery,* a form of bacterial diarrhea. Several well-studied epidemics suggest that about 20 percent of subjects who are B27 positive and experience Shigella dysentery will develop Reiter's syndrome.

It seems likely that no single bacterium causes all cases, but rather that Reiter's syndrome may follow infection with different microorganisms. The Shigella infection is the best established, but some of the venereal cases appear to follow infection with organisms called *Chlamydia* or *Mycoplasma.* Somewhat similar problems are seen after infection with *Yersinia* or *Salmonella* organisms. Thus, different infectious syndromes may precede development of Reiter's syndrome.

This interplay between the genetic predisposition represented by the B27 gene and the necessity for attack by a microorganism provides a fascinating interaction for scientific study. These studies, now being conducted at many medical centers, are likely to lead to major advances in managing Reiter's syndrome over the next several years.

Features

Reiter's disease occurs mostly in men and is episodic, with each episode lasting several weeks to several months. There are frequently recurrences in subsequent years. The arthritis shares many features of ankylosing spondylitis and of psoriatic arthritis.

Like ankylosing spondylitis, the main problem is at the attachment where ligaments and tendons insert into the bone. Thus, involvement of the sacroiliac joints and of the spine is common. Since Reiter's syndrome tends to involve the peripheral parts of the body more than ankylosing spondylitis, a common feature is heel pain, either on the bottom of the heel where the ligaments that form the arch attach or on the back of the heel where the Achilles tendon attaches.

Like psoriatic arthritis, Reiter's syndrome tends to involve the peripheral joints in a random way. Thus, just a few joints are usually involved, and these joints are usually not the same on the two sides of the body. A sausage digit, as described in Chapter 2, is sometimes seen, where involvement of several joints of a toe or finger gives that digit the appearance of a sausage. Usually, in psoriatic arthritis, the upper extremities are involved more than the lower, while with Reiter's syndrome the feet and toes are more frequently involved than are the hands.

Eye problems usually involve only one eye at a time. This may be conjunctivitis ("pink eye") or an inflammation affecting the deeper parts of the eye, causing pain on exposure to bright light or interference with vision.

Discharge from the urethra is the third major feature and usually consists of a clear, watery discharge that does not cause discomfort. While this frequently lasts only a few days or weeks, it may reappear later. It is more apparent in men than in women.

The skin rash occurs only in a few patients, but can help with the diagnosis. The scaling, red skin lesions are most common on the palms and soles and are sometimes not immediately noticed because they don't hurt or itch. Shallow sores of the penis or of the female genital organs may occur; these are also usually painless. Some cases of Reiter's disease with skin involvement resemble psoriatic arthritis, and distinction between the two can be difficult.

X-ray changes usually take several years to develop. Inflammation of the sacroiliac joint, as in ankylosing spondylitis, is common. Stiffening of the spine can also be seen. In distinction to ankylosing spondylitis, Reiter's syndrome frequently involves one side of the body while sparing the other and may skip around from one side to another in different parts of the spine. X-rays of the heels may show bone spurs at the points of attachment where the heel pain is noted.

Laboratory tests are not particularly helpful in diagnosis. The latex test for rheumatoid factor is negative. The antinuclear antibody test is negative. The sedimentation rate is sometimes elevated and sometimes not. The test for the B27 antigen will usually be positive, but this test is not available at many hospitals.

Prognosis

Reiter's syndrome is characterized by an episodic course. Some patients have only one episode and no further recurrences. Or, periods of activity of the disease will alternate with periods of relative inactivity. It is unusual for the arthritis to be crippling, but this can happen.

Problems with the eye can result in loss of sight, usually in just one eye, late in the disease and in a very few cases. The skin problems seldom pose real difficulties and are usually present only a small part of the time.

Those individuals with Reiter's syndrome who do not have the B27 gene probably do a little better than those who have the gene. The first episode usually gives some indication of the disease's future severity; like most forms of arthritis, Reiter's syndrome varies from mild to severe, with most patients doing relatively well.

Treatment

As in ankylosing spondylitis, the most frequent medications used are indomethacin (p. 102) and phenylbutazone (p. 101). In very severe cases, methotrexate (p. 125), azathioprine (p. 125), or other experimental drugs may be required. Corticosteroids such as prednisone are not very helpful and should almost never be used.

Reiter's syndrome is sometimes difficult to treat and may be resistant to all of the anti-inflammatory agents. Sometimes, a few weeks or even months later, a drug that seemed ineffective the first time will prove effective. Hence, when the disease is difficult to control, the physician may periodically rotate drugs to determine which will work the best. Since the disease comes in cycles, control can ultimately be achieved, but it may take disturbingly long to find the right treatment.

Although infections seem to cause Reiter's syndrome, antibiotics do not seem to be an effective treatment. Many physicians have tried tetracycline and other antibiotics, but the results have been very inconsistent.

Eye involvement may require treatment with corticosteroids applied locally. In severe cases, the steroid may be injected into the eye or behind the eye. The skin problems seldom require any treatment. Involvement of the aortic valve, exceedingly rare, may require replacement of that valve surgically.

Surgery for the joints is rarely needed in Reiter's syndrome. Range-of-motion exercises and a judicious balance between rest and graded exercise are important. See instructions for particular joints in Part III.

If you have Reiter's Syndrome, proceed now to Part II, page 87.

Crystal Arthritis:

Inflammation within the Joint Space

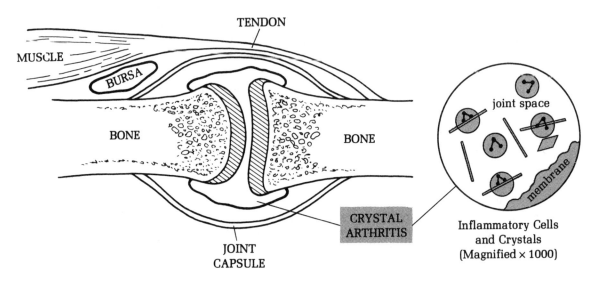

CRYSTAL ARTHRITIS

TENDON

MUSCLE

BURSA

BONE

BONE

joint space

CRYSTAL ARTHRITIS

membrane

Inflammatory Cells
and Crystals
(Magnified × 1000)

JOINT CAPSULE

In Crystal (or Microcrystalline) Arthritis chemical crystals in the joint space cause an inflammation to develop. The inflammation represents the efforts of the body to remove the crystals, but the process is very painful. Gout and Pseudogout are the two most common kinds of crystal arthritis.

GOUT

The word *gout* calls to mind a king, rather red-faced and corpulent, reclining in an easy chair with a very sore foot propped up on a pillow. In fact, gout is a most painful disease and can sometimes result from overindulgence. Many people don't think that gout is arthritis, but it most certainly is. It is the best example of a crystal arthritis, in which the body's reaction to small mineral crystals in the joint space causes a painful illness. The crystals of gout are made up of uric acid and the inflammatory reaction is extremely intense.

Gout crystals cannot develop without an elevated level of uric acid in the body fluids. Unless the fluids are supersaturated, no crystals can form and no reaction can take place. Hence, the condition underlying the disease of gout is called *hyperuricemia*, which simply means "increased uric acid in the blood" and is not a disease at all but just a variation from normal. Hyperuricemia has been related to greater intelligence and to greater tension and anxiety. By itself, the elevated uric acid in the blood does no harm. It is only when the crystals form in the body that trouble can result.

The medical problem of gout has been essentially solved. Dramatic scientific advances have provided adequate treatment for all patients with gout. Drugs such as probenecid, allopurinol, and colchicine are very effective. Yet gout today is treated incorrectly as commonly as it is treated correctly. The drugs are administered to the wrong patients and for the wrong reasons.

Because hyperuricemia is, in part, genetic, there is unlikely to be a cure. However, measures that stop the gout attack and lower the level of uric acid control the disease totally, although the condition will return if these measures are stopped. Science continues to unravel elaborate mysteries of uric acid chemistry, and some forms of gout have already been linked to problems with particular enzymes. So, while further advances in understanding of the disease are likely, the therapy of today is entirely satisfactory and is not likely to be improved on within the foreseeable future.

Features

Gout consists of four stages, beginning with the tendency to develop gout and progressing through the gouty attack to a long-term disease. Many people have the first stage and very few experience the last.

The first stage is called *asymptomatic hyperuricemia*. As the name suggests, this means that the level of uric acid in the blood is raised without any resulting problems. Uric acid levels go up a little in boys at about puberty and in women at about the time of menopause, so sex hormones have some effect on uric-acid level. The levels will go up before an examination at school or at a particularly stressful time of life. Asymptomatic hyperuricemia is defined as having a uric-acid level higher than that of 95 percent of the population. With most tests used today, this means a level higher than about 8 mg%. Asymptomatic hyperuricemia fluctuates somewhat, but tends to persist once it has occurred. Even in those few subjects who go on to the second stage, the period of asymptomatic hyperuricemia usually lasts about 20 years before anything happens.

Acute gouty arthritis, or gout, is the second stage. Here, the body fluids saturated with uric acid have begun to form crystals. The crystals form in the joint fluid and the body reacts with a strong inflammatory attack. Sometimes there is no apparent cause for the attack of gout; other times it happens after surgery, after eating particularly rich foods, after an alcoholic binge, or after an injury to the area. At any rate, the affected part begins to swell and becomes red and painful over a period of a few hours. Soon, the area is too tender to touch; even the touch of bedclothes causes exquisite pain. If not treated, the attack will peak in two or three days and will gradually disappear over about a two-week period. After the attack, the joint and surrounding tissue are entirely normal, until the next attack.

Acute gout affects most commonly the base of the great toe. This form of gout is so common as to have a special name, *podagra.* Next most common is the knee, then the ankle, and then the instep of the foot. Less frequently joints of the upper extremity, particularly the shoulder, wrist, or elbow, may be involved. As a rule, just one joint is involved at a time. Very rarely, two, three, or four joints are involved simultaneously—never more. Patients with a strong tendency toward gout may have five or six attacks a year.

The third, rather simple stage is called *interval gout.* This is really just like the first stage, except that it represents the period between attacks in a patient who has already had an attack of gout. During this stage asymptomatic hyperuricemia is present, but the likelihood of an attack of gout is much greater for the patient who has previously had an attack.

The fourth stage is called *chronic tophaceous gout.* This problem, unlike acute gout, does not come and go. Here, the crystals of uric acid have begun to accumulate in the body, causing deposits of a gritty, chalky material. These deposits are called *tophi.* They can sometimes be seen just under the skin, particularly around the joints and in the ear. They can also grow inside the bone near the joints, causing destruction of the bone. In rare circumstances, they form inside the kidney and can interfere with functioning of the kidney. Kidney stones composed of the uric acid sometimes form.

Doctors generally think of gout as occurring in two types of patients. In the first type, the body makes too much uric acid; the kidneys excrete the uric acid normally into the urine, but can't get rid of it fast enough. In the second type, the body makes a normal amount of uric acid, but the kidneys are unable to get rid of it adequately, so the blood level increases. The first type of gout, with increased production of uric acid, is the more serious and can lead to the problems of tophaceous gout.

The uric-acid test (p. 119) is important to diagnosis; however, as this test is sometimes inaccurate, a doctor may wish to repeat it with another version (called the *uricase* method) that gives a more accurate result. Many doctors will want to measure the amount of uric acid in a 24-hour urine specimen to determine how much uric acid the body is excreting.

Acute gout is one of few diseases that can be diagnosed absolutely accurately. This is done by taking a sample of the joint fluid and looking at it under the microscope. In acute gout, in 95 percent of the cases, the uric-acid crystals can be seen in the joint fluid, surrounded by the body's white cells which are trying frantically to eat them. The crystals can be seen clearly only with polarized light, so polarizing lenses are required.

Prognosis

The overall prognosis for gout is always excellent. No significant problem with health should result from a gouty condition if the patient carefully follows the recommendations of a competent physician. The prognosis varies depending on the stage of the disease.

Asymptomatic hyperuricemia is not a disease at all and very seldom requires treatment. The prognosis does depend on the level of the elevated uric acid; patients with uric-acid levels in the very highest ranges have at least a 50 percent chance of developing an attack of acute gout or of developing a kidney stone. The exact frequency of acute gout or kidney stone is still debated, but it is infrequent except at very high levels of uric acid.

Acute gout will run its course, without treatment, over a couple of weeks. However, with treatment, relief can usually be obtained in just a few hours and the response to treatment is usually dramatic. Thus, acute gout requires treatment as soon as possible in the course of the attack.

During the interval between attacks, the frequency of previous attacks is the best guide to their recurrence. After a single first attack, only half of the patients will have a second. Thereafter, recurrence becomes the rule rather than the exception, and most patients will have additional attacks. These usually can be prevented by appropriate treatment.

In tophaceous gout, stage 4, the condition slowly progresses until some damage is caused to the joints or the kidneys. With treatment, the tophi slowly dissolve and are excreted through the urine as uric acid. If the tophi are large, they may leave some destruction behind, but usually there is healing. Hence, while we don't like to see tophaceous gout (and see it very rarely now), even this stage can be effectively treated.

There is still controversy about the effects of elevated levels of uric acid on the kidney. Theoretically, damage could occur, but in practice we can't detect any significant problem. Any kidney disease due to uric acid would progress very slowly over a period of years and should be easily treatable until very advanced. Hence, most doctors feel that kidney tests should be performed every few years in patients with elevated uric acid levels, but that treatment is not required in the absence of an actual problem.

Treatment

To some extent, gout is a disease of life-style. It is affected by body weight, by diet, and by alcohol. Thus, it can be treated by a more rational life-style, including a reasonable body weight, a good exercise level, and a diet that excludes high-uric-acid foods such as liver, pancreas, and brain. Strict diets are very seldom needed. Intake of a large amount of fluid will increase urine flow and assist in removing uric acid from the body. Alkalinizing the urine will result in faster elimination of uric acid, since uric acid is more soluble when the urine is alkaline (basic) than when it is acid.

Moreover, a lot of elevated-uric-acid problems are caused by drugs, and stopping those drugs or switching to less bothersome ones can alleviate the problem entirely. Most notorious are water pills or diuretics (particularly the thiazide diuretics such as Diuril or Esidrix), but many other drugs also can cause elevation of uric acid. This is just another reason to manage your life with as few drugs as possible.

Medical treatment is the mainstay of management. Selection of the particular drug depends on the stage of the disease. With asymptomatic hyperuricemia, no treatment is required and you should question a treatment recommendation if you are not having problems. To be rational at all, treatment of an elevated uric acid level must be continued for life, and in a typical patient with treatment begun at age thirty-five, the cost and compound interest on the drugs used may exceed $20,000! The treatment will involve 38,325 pills! For most people, any value received from such treatment will not justify its cost, and some patients will experience side effects that will increase the cost yet more.

Acute gout is treated with agents that block the inflammatory reaction, and a number of drugs do this effectively. Colchicine, the traditional favorite, can be given by mouth or by vein (p. 120). Its problem: it causes diarrhea when given by mouth and the diarrhea can be quite severe. Phenylbutazone (p. 101) is another frequent choice and is extremely effective, with very rare side effects. Indomethacin (p. 102) and other anti-inflammatory agents are frequently effective. And, ACTH injections or corticosteroids are favored by a few physicians, although not by most. Any of these modalities may be used; patients who have compared several different treatments tend to prefer phenylbutazone by mouth or colchicine by vein.

In the interval between attacks, a drug may be given to reduce the uric acid level. Usually these agents are not started during the attack, because they unfortunately can prolong the acute attack. Probenecid (p. 121) and allopurinol (p. 122) are the two most frequent choices; probenecid is usually preferred unless the 24-hour urine test shows excretion of a large amount of uric acid, in which case allopurinol is often chosen. With both of these drugs, low dose colchicine also is frequently used to prevent attacks. The colchicine dose can be low enough so that diarrhea does not occur, and it is effective in reducing the number of new attacks. Meanwhile, the excess uric acid in the body is being slowly eliminated through the urine.

With chronic tophaceous gout (stage 4), an agent to increase excretion or decrease production of uric acid is essential. Probenecid or allopurinol will always be used. Colchicine also may be used to limit the frequency of acute attacks. In severe cases, probenecid and allopurinol may be used together. Because of effective treatment, chronic tophaceous gout is a vanishing disease.

If your problem is gout, proceed now to Part II, page 87.

PSEUDOGOUT

Pseudogout is a name both colorful and apt for this recently recognized form of arthritis. The name suggests that the disease is similar to gout, as is the case, and *pseudogout* is much less cumbersome than the alternative names *calcium pyrophosphate crystal deposition disease* or *chondrocalcinosis*. These names are also useful in that they provide a summary description of the major disease features. As in gout, crystals in the joint space cause an intense inflammatory reaction that results in redness and pain in the joint. In this case, the crystals are not uric acid but are pyrophosphate crystals. They are deposited into the joint space from the nearby cartilage, where they can be seen on X-ray. *Chondro* means "cartilage"; hence the name *chondrocalcinosis* refers to calcium in the cartilage of the joint. These crystals are preformed and discharged into the joint, rather than forming in the joint space as they do in gout. A similar syndrome occurs with other minerals that can form crystals, such as hydroxyapatite, but uric acid and calcium pyrophosphate are the two main offenders. The calcium does *not* come from drinking too much milk, and diet will neither help nor hurt this condition.

Pseudogout is much more a disease of aging than is gout, and the calcium accumulates slowly in the cartilage over a long period. In patients with rare metabolic disease, such as parathyroid disease or hemochromatosis, the condition may occur earlier in life. Generally, however, pseudogout is a disease of the later years.

Features

Typically, a patient with pseudogout will have acute attacks of crystal arthritis much like gout. The calcium crystals excite a less violent response than do uric-acid crystals, so pain is not always as severe, but the discharge of crystals may continue, causing the attack to last longer. Hence, many patients with pseudogout don't have as clear a pattern of attacks separated by symptom-free intervals. They may have problems more or less continuously.

The average age of a patient at first attack is about 70 years. Males and females are affected in approximately similar frequencies (unlike gout, which tends to affect men more frequently than women). The joint most often involved is the knee, followed by the wrists and the ankles. More often than in gout, several joints may be involved at one time. Attacks may be brought on by stress or surgery, as in gout, but overeating or the eating of rich foods is not related to attacks.

Often there is some cartilage degeneration in the affected joints, and the tendency of this condition to last for weeks or months may be partly related to the associated degenerative disease.

Laboratory tests are not very helpful. Blood tests are usually entirely normal. But X-ray findings are very important. On the X-ray, calcium can be seen in the cartilage of the affected joints and sometimes in other joints. And, if the joint fluid is removed through a needle, the crystals of calcium pyrophosphate can be seen in the joint fluid. These rather square crystals contrast with the long, needle-like crystals seen in gout.

Together, the finding of calcium in the cartilage on X-ray and the identification of calcium crystals in the joint fluid establish the diagnosis of pseudogout.

Prognosis

The prognosis for pseudogout is good. Very seldom does crippling result, although over half of pseudogout patients will have recurrent attacks and many will experience some degree of sustained pain. Attacks may continue for a long time. They tend to get better for a while and then worse for a while; most patients are able to carry on quite normal activities despite the problems.

Pseudogout seems to affect only the joints, so patients otherwise feel entirely well. There is no involvement of any other organs and thus no truly serious threats to health. The condition does not seem to be genetically related so there is no particular risk to family members.

Treatment

Treatment is helpful but not as dramatically so as with gout. The most effective drugs are indomethacin (p. 102), phenylbutazone (p. 101), or other anti-inflammatory agents. Frequently, these agents must be taken rather steadily to continue the relief. Colchicine, which is consistently effective in gout, helps some people with pseudogout, but does not seem to help others.

Careful exercises and graded activities for the involved joints and preservation of normal living styles are important. (See the discussions in Part III for specific instructions.) Weight control is particularly crucial if the weight-bearing joints are involved by the pseudogout. Techniques of joint protection, as noted in Chapter 19, are helpful.

Obviously, the drugs for gout that control uric-acid level, such as allopurinol and probenecid, should not be expected to help pseudogout, and they don't. The uric-acid level is normal in pseudogout. Surgery is very seldom required, but we have seen patients who eventually needed replacement of a knee of even a hip. In general, treatment should be mild and conservative.

Strong agents such as cortisone and its derivatives are not helpful and carry serious hazards, although steroid injections into the joint are sometimes helpful.

If your problem is pseudogout, proceed now to Part II, page 87.

Infections:

Infection in the Joint Space

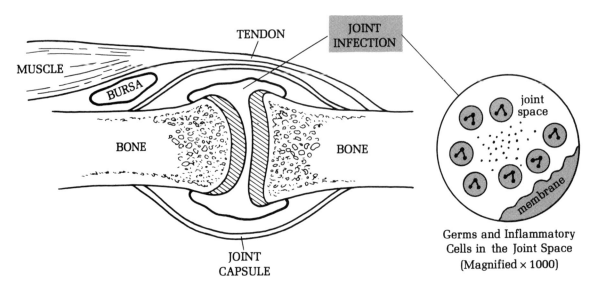

JOINT INFECTION

TENDON

JOINT INFECTION

MUSCLE

BURSA

BONE

BONE

joint space

membrane

JOINT CAPSULE

Germs and Inflammatory Cells in the Joint Space (Magnified × 1000)

If bacteria lodge and grow within the joint space, an "infectious" arthritis is present. This kind of arthritis requires antibiotics for its treatment, and treatment represents an emergency. The infection can spread to other parts of the body or can destroy the involved joint.

The most common bacteria causing this problem are the staphylococcus, the gonococcus, and the tuberculosis germ.

The single hot joint is an emergency and needs immediate attention, because it might be a bacterial infection. When bacteria invade the joint space, the joint becomes a giant boil filled with pus. Warm, red skin surrounds the joint and there is swelling with considerable pain.

Almost every type of bacteria seems at some time or another to have caused an infectious arthritis, but the staphylococcus infection is possibly the most serious. Further, staphylococcus and gonococcus (discussed in the next section) infections are the two most common.

How do bacteria get into the joint? Sometimes they get in through the bloodstream as part of an infection elsewhere in the body. Sometimes the initial infection may not be noticed, but a few bacteria may lodge in the joint while passing by. More rarely, bacteria are introduced by a previous injection into the knee or by a direct injury. Infection is a rare complication of joint injection, and can happen even with the most careful physician and best techniques. The germs tend to lodge in previously damaged joints, so patients with arthritis are more likely than others to develop an infectious arthritis. A single hot joint appearing in a patient with an underlying arthritis is just as serious as a hot joint in a patient with no previous arthritis. Some arthritis patients are more susceptible because of lowered resistance due to a serious disease or because of resistance-reducing drugs. In many cases, no one knows how the bacteria got into the joint—they just mysteriously appear.

Staphylococcal germs vary, and some are worse than others. With a particularly bad strain of staph, the joint may be seriously damaged in as little as one or two days; with less destructive organisms, it may take several weeks for damage to occur. Staph infection of a joint is a serious disease that can result in joint destruction.

Features

Bacterial infection of the joint, with staphylococcus as the best example, is acute. It develops over a period of hours to days. The arthritis is severe and the affected joint is red, warm, and swollen. A staphylococcal infection of a joint is in no way subtle—symptoms are pronounced and easily discernible.

Usually only one joint is involved, although on occasion two or three or even four may be involved. Most frequently, the knee is the infected joint. The ankle, the wrist, the shoulder, the elbow, and the hips are also relatively common. Other joints are affected less frequently. Thus, infections tend to occur in the largest joints of the body.

Since this is an infection, there may be fever and the patient may feel generally ill. The white blood count may be elevated and the sedimentation rate may be raised. Both of these tests may be normal in other cases. Other blood tests are not helpful, except for a culture of the blood, which is used to identify the offending bacterium.

X-rays may show bony destruction at the joint after a few days or a few months, if treatment has not been early enough. The changes revealed by X-ray lag behind the disease's progress, however, so the X-ray is not as helpful as might be supposed.

The key test is removal of fluid from the joint, examination of this fluid under the microscope, and culture for bacteria. The joint fluid will look like pus and will be swarming with polymorphonuclear white cells trying to fight the infection. The bacteria will be seen in the joint fluid and sometimes inside the cells that are trying to engulf them. The culture, one to two days later, will usually grow out of the germ and permit a positive identification. The joint fluid test also allows the doctor to eliminate the possibility of gout, which is the most frequently mistaken diagnosis.

Prognosis

Staphylococcal infection of the joint, if identified and treated properly, has an excellent prognosis. In some two weeks the joint should be much better, although fluid may accumulate for yet another week or so. There should be no long-term bad results of any kind. If treatment is delayed, destruction of the bone and seeding of the infection to other parts of body may occur, with ominous consequences. Without any treatment, staphylococcal joint infection would be a fatal disease most of the time.

Relatively rarely, the bone next to the joint may become infected, causing an osteomyelitis. This can be a serious complication requiring long-term antibiotic treatment or surgery.

Treatment

A high "index of suspicion" and prompt diagnosis are the keys to good results in treating staph infections. The proper antibiotics must be started as quickly as possible and in adequate doses. Except in patients who are allergic to penicillin, one of the penicillinlike antibiotics will be used. Initial treatment is by intravenous injection, and almost all doctors hospitalize patients with staphylococcal joint infections, at least during the early stages of treatment. If a great deal of fluid is accumulating, it may be removed from the joint with a needle every day or every several days. If this is still not adequate, surgical drainage of the extra pus is performed by some physicians. The antibiotic should be continued for at least ten days to two weeks, and often for six weeks. Some follow-up is needed to insure that the infection is gone and that there is no related infection in the bone.

This form of arthritis can be cured—or it can be fatal. Cure requires that you consult a competent physician promptly, so that appropriate treatment may be started. The single hot joint is a signal to see the physician today.

If your problem is staphylococcal arthritis, proceed now to Part II, page 87.

We think of gonorrhea as a venereal disease. Sometimes it is called GC, or clap, or gonorrhea, or the whites, or some other picturesque name. It is less well known that gonorrhea can cause an arthritis called *gonococcal arthritis*. This is an infectious arthritis in which the gonococcal bacteria grows in the joint space. This is one of the most common causes of arthritis in young women between the ages of 15 and 25.

During a genital infection with the gonococcal bacteria, the bacteria may travel in the blood to the joint space. The gonococcal bacteria is unusual in that it grows well only in the particular parts of the body, such as the urethra or the joints. The body defenses are good against the GC organism; even bloodstream infections that have seeded the joints can occasionally be overcome by body defenses alone, without the aid of antibiotics.

Features

For the most part, gonococcal arthritis is a disease of young women. It occurs ten times as frequently in women as in men. There appear to be several reasons for this. In women, the gonorrhea infection of the vagina and cervix may not be noticed by the patient, whereas a man almost always notices discharge from the penis. So, in women, the infection may remain untreated until a menstrual period comes. During the menstrual period, the bacteria can get into the bloodstream from the uterus and can move through the bloodstream to other areas of the body. Most cases of gonococcal arthritis begin during the menstrual cycle.

Gonococcal arthritis affects one to several joints, but does not affect many joints at the same time. The most common joint is the knee. Second most common is the wrist, with a tendency to involve the back of the wrist around the tendons that operate the fingers. This is called *tenosynovitis*. The arthritis caused by gonococcal infection will seem to move from one joint to another and usually will not be the same on both sides of the body. For example, a right knee, a left wrist, and a right ankle may be affected.

The skin can provide important clues to the presence of a gonococcal infection. Little blisters on a red base may be found, often only one or two over the entire body. These blisters contain the gonococcal bacteria and are evidence that the infection has moved through the bloodstream and might be infecting the joints.

In men, a white discharge from the penis is almost always present. In women, a vaginal discharge and sometimes fever or abdominal pain may be present. Infection of the rectum or of the mouth may occur with the gonococcal bacteria. Physicians will usually culture the various body fluids that may be infected to locate the bacteria. The discharge from the penis or the vagina is usually culture positive, but a culture from the joint fluid is frequently negative. This may indicate that the body is already in the process of cleaning up that infection.

No other laboratory findings are positive, with the exception of an elevated white count indicating infection or perhaps a mildly elevated sedimentation rate. There usually will not be any X-ray changes.

Prognosis

Gonococcal arthritis clears up without any damage if it is diagnosed promptly and treated properly. It may take several days to get the joints all calmed down and fluid may reaccumulate in some joints for several weeks, but ultimately all symptoms clear up and there are no residual problems unless the patient is reinfected.

Even before antibiotic treatment was available, most people did not suffer disability from gonococcal arthritis. However, with the potential for serious complications and with curative treatment available, it is essential that all patients be promptly diagnosed and treated.

Treatment

The key to treatment is antibiotics. Usually the antibiotic will be penicillin or one of its derivatives (unless the patient is allergic to penicillin). Many physicians hospitalize the patient for the first few days and many administer the antibiotics through the vein to ensure that the antibiotic directly attacks the bacteria site. On some occasions, the joint will be drained of excess fluid and, in rare instances, antibiotics may be put directly into an infected joint. Usually this is not necessary.

It must be remembered that gonococcal arthritis comes from a venereal disease. Treatment includes not only the patient but also the sexual contacts of the patient, who may be unknowingly spreading the disease to additional persons. If you are the patient, it is critical that you help your sexual partners by ensuring that they know about the disease and that they go for adequate treatment. Help is readily available at the local county health department.

If your problem is gonococcal arthritis, proceed now to Part II, page 87.

TUBERCULOSIS (TB)

Tuberculosis of the joint is rare. For that matter, tuberculosis itself is now relatively rare. But arthritis caused by a tuberculosis bacterium is typical of slow, less obvious infections of the joint space, so we describe it here. Not only the tuberculosis bacterium but also various kinds of fungus, such as histoplasmosis of coccidioidomycosis, may result in the same sort of slow, long-term infection.

As many as 50 percent of patients with arthritis due to tuberculosis do not have tuberculosis of the lungs. Tuberculous arthritis may develop for months or even years before diagnosis is made. Treatment of the joint problem is usually not difficult, but, because it is rare, neither doctor nor patient may think of it.

Don't worry too much about having tuberculosis of the joint, because it is unusual. But, bear in mind that occasionally a long-term swelling of a single joint may be due to infection, in addition to the short-term, red, hot process that we usually associate with infection.

Features

In one study, tuberculous arthritis was not diagnosed for an average of 19 months, and in one patient the process of making the diagnosis took 12 years. Usually, the knee or the hip is involved. The tuberculosis organism needs a large space to grow in, so the smaller joints are generally not infected. Once in a while, we will see arthritis caused by tuberculosis or a fungus in a small joint of the hand or foot.

Usually, just one joint is involved. Arthritis is seen in far less than one percent of patients with tuberculosis.

Tuberculosis of the spine used to be called Pott's disease. It was fairly common at one time, although in recent years cases have been few and far between. The key feature of a Pott's abscess (or of a tuberculous arthritis of a peripheral joint) is that it is a "cold" abscess. Unlike bacterial infection (for example, boils), tuberculosis and fungus do not excite a very violent inflammation and the affected area is usually about the same temperature as the surrounding tissues, instead of being hot and red.

Diagnosis can be made by culture of the joint fluid in 80 percent of the cases. A biopsy of the lining tissue of the joint, the synovium, will be positive in most of the rest. Some scientists have thought that a low glucose (blood sugar) in the synovial space is common in tuberculous arthritis, others have found this less frequently.

X-rays taken over a long period of time may show some destruction of the bone next to the joint infection. The bone changes usually take years to develop, and it is unlikely that any will be present until after a number of months have passed.

Laboratory tests commonly positive in other forms of arthritis will usually be negative in tuberculous arthritis.

Prognosis

In tuberculous arthritis, prognosis depends on the time of diagnosis. If the diagnosis is early and the tuberculosis in other parts of the body is not causing major problems, the prognosis is essentially complete recovery. The tuberculous infection can be cured and the patient will have no disability. If diagnosis is delayed and there has been destruction of the cartilage, then there may be some disability. Occasionally, in the presence of severe tuberculosis in other organs, even good treatment will not prevent death.

Treatment

Suspicion of the disease and the making of a correct diagnosis are crucial. After diagnosis, the joint fluid may be drained periodically. Antituberculosis medications are given by mouth for from two to three years. Improvement is generally noted within the first few weeks and is complete within a few months. Treatment is continued longer than this to prevent recurrence.

If your problem is tuberculous arthritis, proceed to Part II, page 87.

VIRAL INFECTIONS

The joints can be affected by other infectious agents, including viruses. These problems are minor, unusual, and last only a few days or weeks. German measles (Rubella) can cause such a reaction, as can immunization against German measles. Hepatitis can do the same. A new kind of arthritis, Lyme arthritis, involves an infection of unknown type transmitted by a tick bite.

If your problem is viral arthritis, proceed now to Part II, page 87.

Cartilage Degeneration:

Wearing Out of the Joint Gristle

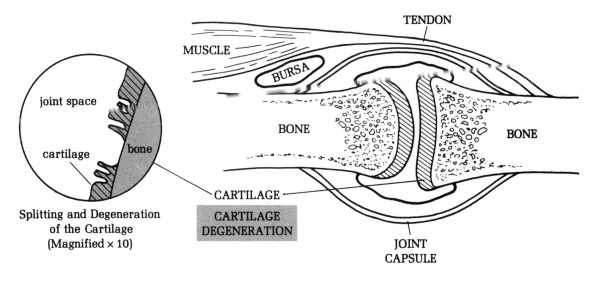

CARTILAGE DEGENERATION

TENDON

MUSCLE

BURSA

joint space

BONE

BONE

cartilage

bone

CARTILAGE

Splitting and Degeneration
of the Cartilage
(Magnified × 10)

CARTILAGE
DEGENERATION

JOINT
CAPSULE

The cartilage or gristle which absorbs the shock of joint motion can wear down and degenerate, leaving two surfaces of bone in contact with each other. The cartilage first frays and splits, and eventually can almost disappear. There is little or no inflammation. This type of arthritis is called osteoarthritis, degenerative joint disease, OA, DJD, or osteoarthrosis.

OSTEOARTHRITIS (OSTEOARTHROSIS, OA, DEGENERATIVE JOINT DISEASE, DJD)

This is the kind of arthritis that almost everybody gets. It is a practically universal problem that increases with age. It is not as responsive to medical treatment as we might like. Fortunately, osteoarthritis usually is a mild condition. The majority of people with osteoarthritis don't have any pain or stiffness and the majority of the remainder have only occasional problems. Hence, osteoarthritis is a much more benign form of arthritis than those discussed previously. In other words, the changes in the skeleton that occur with age are inevitable, but they cause symptoms in relatively few people and severe symptoms in very few.

The tissue involved in osteoarthritis is the cartilage. This is the gristle material that faces the ends of the bones and forms the surface of the joint on both sides. Gristle is tough, somewhat elastic, and very durable. The cartilage or gristle does not have a blood supply, so it gets its oxygen and nutrition from the surrounding joint fluid. In this it is aided by being elastic and by being able to absorb fluid. When we use a joint, the pressure expresses fluid and waste products out of the cartilage and, when the pressure is relieved, the fluid seeps back, together with oxygen and nutrients. Hence, the health of the cartilage depends on use of the joint. Over many years, the cartilage may become frayed and may even wear away entirely. When this happens, the bone surface on one side of the joint grates against the bone on the other side of the joint, providing a much less elastic joint surface. With time, the opposing bony surfaces may become polished, a process called *eburnation*. As this happens, the joint may again move more smoothly and cause less discomfort.

Osteoarthritis is sometimes called osteoarthrosis. The difference between these two long terms has to do with the question of inflammation. *Itis* denotes inflammation, and with cartilage degeneration very little inflammation is to be found. Hence, some experts prefer the term osteoarthrosis, which does not imply inflammation.

There are three common forms of osteoarthritis, and many people have some of each type. The first and mildest causes knobby enlargement of the finger joints. The end joints of the fingers become bony and the hands begin to assume the appearance we associate with old age. The other joints of the fingers also may be involved. This kind of arthritis (or arthrosis) usually causes little difficulty beyond the cosmetic. There may be some stiffness.

The second form of osteoarthrosis involves the spine. Bony growths appear on the spine in the neck region or in the low back. Usually the bony growths are associated with some narrowing of the space between the vertebrae. This time the disk rather than cartilage is the material that becomes frayed. Changes in the spine begin early in life in almost all of us, but cause symptoms relatively seldom.

The third-form of osteoarthrosis involves the weight-bearing joints, almost always the hips and knees. These problems can be quite severe. It is possible to have all three kinds of osteoarthrosis or any two of them, but often a patient will have only one.

Patients who have had fractures near a joint or have a congenital malformation at a joint seem to develop osteoarthritis in those joints at an earlier age. On the other hand, the usual description of this arthritis as "wear and tear" is not accurate. While excessive wear and tear on the joint can theoretically result in damage, activity helps the joint remain supple and lubricated and this tends to cancel out the theoretical bad effects.

At any rate, careful studies of people who regularly put a lot of stress on joints (such as individuals who operate pneumatic drills or run long distances on hard paved surfaces) have been unable to establish a relationship between these activities and the development of arthritis. Hence, intensive activity does not predispose you to arthritis any more than intensive activity predisposes you to heart disease. In fact, the very opposite may be true.

Features

The bony knobs that form around the end joints of the finger are called *Heberden's nodes* after the British doctor who first described them. In the middle joints of the fingers, similar knobs can be found. Usually, the bony enlargement occurs slowly over a period of years and is not even noticed by the patient. In most cases, all of the fingers are involved more or less equally.

There is an interesting variation of osteoarthritis in which the bony swelling occurs over only three or four weeks in a single finger joint. The sudden swelling will cause redness and soreness until the process is complete; then, it will stop hurting altogether. This syndrome is seen in women in their forties, earlier than the more usual form of osteoarthritis. These patients frequently have other family members with the same problem. This "familial" form of osteoarthrosis doesn't really seem very much worse over the long run, but one joint after another may suddenly develop a bony knob for a short period of time.

Osteoarthrosis of the spine doesn't cause symptoms unless there is pressure on one of the nerves or irritation of some of the other structures of the back. In Chapter 8, the section on low back pain describes these problems. If someone tells you that you have arthritis in your spine, don't assume that the pain you feel is necessarily related to that arthritis. Most people with X-rays showing arthritis of the spine don't have any problem at all.

Osteoarthritis of the weight-bearing joints, particularly the hip and knee, develops slowly and often involves both sides of the body. Pain in the joint may remain fairly constant or may wax and wane for a period of years. In severe cases, walking may be difficult or even impossible. Fluid may accumulate in the affected joint, giving it a swollen appearance, or a knee may wobble a bit when weight is placed on it. Usually, in the knee, the osteoarthrosis will affect the inner or the outer half of the joint more than the other; this may result in the leg becoming bowed and cause difficulty in walking.

X-rays are important in evaluating osteoarthritis, although both doctor and patient have to realize that X-ray findings are far more common than symptoms. The two major findings on the X-ray are narrowing of the joint space and the presence of bony spurs. X-rays pass right through cartilage. Hence, in a normal joint, the X-ray looks as though the two bones are separated by a space. In reality, the apparent space is filled with cartilage. As the cartilage is frayed, the apparent joint space on the X-ray narrows until the two bones may touch each other. *Osteophytes*, or spurs, are little bony growths that appear alongside the places where the cartilage has degenerated. It is as though the body is trying to react to a cartilage problem by providing more surface area for the joint, so as to distribute the weight more evenly. At any rate, the bony growth provides a larger joint surface, although the new bone is not covered by cartilage. In addition, X-rays can sometimes show the holes through which the nerves pass and indicate whether these holes are narrowed or not.

In contrast to X-rays, blood tests aren't very helpful in osteoarthritis. There's nothing wrong with the rest of the body, so all tests are normal.

Prognosis

Prognosis is usually good for osteoarthritis. When one think of an aging process, one tends to thinks of a progressive condition that continues to get worse and worse. This is not necessarily the case. Osteoarthritis may get worse for a time and then become stable for a long period. A joint that has lost its cartilage may not function well at first, but, with use, the bone may be molded and polished so that a smooth and more functional joint develops. Even in the worst cases, osteoarthritis progresses slowly. You have lots of time to think about what kinds of treatment are likely to help. If a surgical decision is needed, you have ample time to consider whether you want an operation or not. Crippling from osteoarthritis is relatively rare and most individuals with osteoarthritis remain essentially free of symptoms.

Treatment

Joints should be exercised through their full range of motion several times a day. If weight-bearing joints are involved, body weight should be kept under control. Obesity accelerates the rate of damage to the diseased joint. The most helpful exercises seem to be swimming and walking—activities that are easy, can be gradually increased, and are smooth rather than jerky. Exercise should be regular, and should not hurt much. Thus, if you start getting some osteoarthritis, it is not a signal to begin to tone down your life, but rather to develop a sensible, regular exercise program to strengthen the bones and ligaments surrounding the affected joints and to preserve mobility in joints that are developing spurs.

Drug therapy is much less important. We use it to control the discomfort to a certain extent. Aspirin (p. 98) in moderate doses (or acetaminophen) is frequently helpful. Indomethacin (p. 102) and other anti-inflammatory drugs (p. 100) may be helpful for some people, particularly if the osteoarthritis is in the hip or the knee. I avoid codeine and strong pain pills because pain is a signal to the body that helps protect a diseased joint; it is important that this signal is received. The next section describes the kinds of arthritis that can follow when pain is suppressed too vigorously.

Frequently some kinds of devices can assist. A cane may be helpful; less commonly, crutches are needed. Occasionally special shoes or lifts on one side of the foot may be helpful.

Most physicians believe that osteoarthritis in the symptomatic form may be prevented to a large extent by good health habits. If you are active, maintain a lean body weight, exercise your muscles and joints regularly so as to nourish cartilage, and let your common sense tell you when you've overdone and something hurts, your joints should last a long time. Like exercise of the heart muscle, exercise of the muscles and joints provides reserves for the occasional strenuous activities we all encounter. Exercise builds strong tissues that last a long time.

Injection of osteoarthritic joints with corticosteroids (p. 106) is occasionally helpful, as is removal of some fluid from an involved joint. Unfortunately, injections often don't help much, since there isn't much inflammation to be suppressed. Injections should not be frequently repeated because the injection of cortisone may damage the cartilage and the bone.

Surgery can be dramatically effective for patients with severe osteoarthritis of the weight-bearing joints. The total-hip-replacement operation (p. 131) is the most important operation yet devised for any form of arthritis. Essentially all patients are free of pain after the surgery and many walk normally and engage in normal activities. The total knee replacement (p. 131) is a more recent operation that already gives far better results than knee surgery available just a few years ago. Surgery is not urgent, and you and your doctor will want to decide the point at which the discomfort or the limitation on your walking has become sufficiently great so that the discomfort, the costs, and the small risk associated with the operation are warranted.

If your problem is osteoarthritis, proceed now to Part II, page 87.

JOINTS WITHOUT NERVES (NEUROPATHIC JOINTS)

Although this kind of arthritis is rare, I include it here to indicate the problems that can arise from the relief of pain and to illustrate the principal features of joint protection.

A joint without a nerve supply is spectacularly affected. Cartilage degenerates, bone fractures and distorts, and the joint becomes all but useless. This may take only a few months or a few years. Such joints are often called *Charcot joints,* after the physician who first described them in syphilis.

What connection does this incredible arthritis have with the absence of a nerve supply to the joint? The answer is that normal activities impose tremendous stresses across our joints, but these forces are cushioned by nervous reflexes of which we are not even aware. If you were to jump from a two-foot-high stool and land on a hard surface with your knees locked, the stress across your knee joint would reach several thousand pounds and you might be injured. On the other hand, your joints can tolerate a much higher jump quite readily if the fall is anticipated with bent knees and just the right amount of muscle tension at the time of impact. When we walk or climb stairs, the same thing happens in miniature. Potentially large stresses are absorbed by cushioning actions that require unconscious nervous reflexes. Tiny fibers in the joint and in the limbs tell the brain the position of the limb, and the brain then feeds back nerve impulses that prepare the joint for the next motion or impact. If these reflex nervous arcs are not present because of disease, the joint is quickly destroyed.

In syphilis affecting the nervous system, these reflex arcs may be destroyed. And with certain other diseases of the nervous system, the reflexes can be decreased. All of these conditions are very rare and you don't need to begin worrying about having any of them.

The importance of this discussion is in discovering the importance of pain. Pain is probably the body's single most important defense mechanism. It tells us when something is wrong. In the case of the joints, pain often tells us not to use a particular joint so much, to give it a rest for awhile. The nerve fibers that tell the brain about position are not exactly the same as those that tell about pain, but they are closely related and they are affected by the same kinds of drugs. If you block these reflexes by using too many pain-killers, you act to destroy your joints and to prevent your body from helping you minimize the damage. By causing more damage to the joint, you cause more future pain for yourself, so that the drug giving you temporary pain relief may actually be increasing the amount of pain you will have during your life.

Features

Charcot joints usually affect the knees, one or both, although other weight-bearing joints may be affected. The affected joint is massively swollen, distorted, and unstable. In the leg below the affected joint there is loss of nerve connections, and the physician can find a defect in pain and position perception. The X-rays show loss of cartilage, new bone growth, and frequently fractures at the joint. There are no laboratory test abnormalities in these conditions except those of the underlying disease.

Prognosis

These are severe forms of arthritis, and they usually will progress to serious disability, particularly at the knee. The prognosis is that of the disease that caused the nerve problem, such as syphilis or diabetes.

The underlying disease may be treated effectively if it is syphilis and to some extent if it is diabetes. However, the nerves will not regenerate after treatment of the disease and the joint problem may continue to get worse.

Protection of the joints with crutches or a cane and limited use of the joints are important. Drugs do not help much. Surgery is only rarely attempted and only moderately successful. Artificial joints won't work very well here because of the pounding they take, but fusion of the joint can sometimes help.

If your problem is neuropathic joints, proceed now to Part II, page 87.

Muscle Inflammation:

Inflammation Among Muscle Fibers

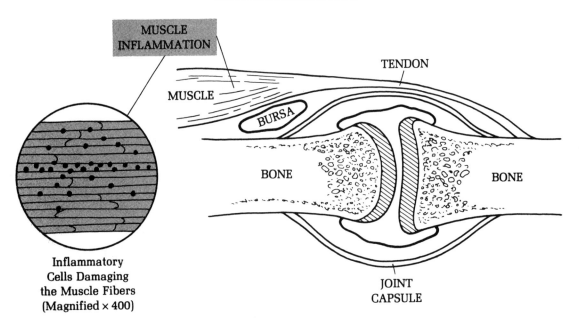

MUSCLE INFLAMMATION

Inflammatory
Cells Damaging
the Muscle Fibers
(Magnified × 400)

Near the joint, the muscles may become inflamed. Here, in polymyositis or dermatomyositis, the inflammatory cells may be seen between and injuring the muscle fibers. In polymyalgia rheumatica the muscles are also involved but the inflammation is in the small blood vessels and is harder to see under the microscope.

When an older person develops severe aching of the muscles, it may be polymalgia rheumatica. This is the most newly recognized major kind of rheumatism. It is a serious condition, but the treatment for it is extremely effective. Hence, it is important to know a little bit about it.

Let's take a look at those long words. The prefix *poly* means "many." The root *my* in the middle of the word means "muscle." The ending *algia* denotes "pain." So, the first long word means "pain in many muscles." The second word *rheumatica* just tells us redundantly that the aching and pain are those we often associate with the rather vague term *rheumatism*.

This syndrome was recognized in the United States in the late 1960s. The cause is unknown, but the pain and disability seem related to inflammation of the small blood vessels that supply the muscles. So, it is probably an *arteritis*—that is, an arterial inflammation—rather than a muscle disease, but it is listed here because the muscle aching is the major feature. It is not related to polymyositis, which involves inflammation of the muscle itself, discussed next.

Because the condition is so serious and the treatment so effective, early detection, diagnosis, and treatment are important. The disease is unusual, but by no means rare. Probably one in several hundred people will experience it.

Features

Polymyalgia rheumatica causes muscle aching in persons over the age of 50 years. It involves principally the muscles of the neck and shoulder regions, frequently with pain and aching in the hip areas also. The average age of patients is close to 70 years. The onset may be gradual or may occur over just a few days. Morning stiffness (see problem 2, Part III) can be pronounced in some patients.

If not diagnosed and treated early, the condition may get worse and may even resemble cancer. Patients may be tired, have low fevers for a long time, and lose significant amounts of weight, even as much as 30 or 40 pounds. There can be a synovitis in some patients, so the joints as well as the muscles ache.

The artery inflammation found in some patients may affect the arteries of the temples on the side of the skull. There may be pain or visible redness over these arteries and they may hurt when pressed. Using the affected muscles, as in using the arm repeatedly or in chewing a thick steak, may cause pain due to inadequacy of blood supply. Rarely, the artery to the eye can be affected, causing blindness in that eye. This is the most serious complication of the disease. When artery inflammation is found, this disease is potentially more severe and is called *giant-cell arteritis*.

In the laboratory, the erythrocyte sedimentation rate (ESR) (p. 136) is greatly elevated. Indeed, this test is higher in polymyalgia rheumatica than in any other disease. Additionally, the level of *fibrinogen*, a soluble protein in the blood, may be raised and the patient is often anemic, sometimes severely.

Biopsies of the arteries are sometimes helpful for diagnosis, but biopsy of the muscle shows surprisingly little damage under the microscope. A biopsy of the temporal artery can sometimes prove the diagnosis of giant-cell arteritis.

There are no X-ray changes characteristic of polymyalgia rheumatica.

Prognosis

Without treatment, this condition appears to last three to five years on the average, gradually disappearing thereafter. During that period, all patients will have been very symptomatic and a few will have lost vision in one or both eyes.

With treatment, on the other hand, the patient is immediately well, typically within two days of beginning treatment. Blindness after treatment is exceedingly rare and complications from treatment are unusual.

Treatment

The cornerstone of treatment is corticosteroid medication. Usually the drug chosen is prednisone (p. 108), and it is started at a medium or high dosage depending on the severity of the case. It is then rapidly decreased to lower doses which must be maintained for some time. Prednisone is typically required for eighteen months to three years, occasionally longer. The prednisone does not cure the disease, but is successful in entirely eliminating the symptoms.

Usually, the increase in activity afforded by the prednisone is so substantial that it makes up for any minor side effects that might occur. There does seem to be a slight tendency for patients on prednisone to develop the shingles and some patients may suffer some osteoporosis or softening of the bones.

The response to treatment is absolutely dramatic. Polymyalgia rheumatica frequently affects individuals who have been active throughout their lives. These patients are very disturbed by their inability to engage in their favorite activities. A patient who loves to play golf, for example, and has been unable to play for the past six months because of pain in the shoulders and neck is likely to become depressed and discouraged. Usually, patients will suggest that it must be "old age" catching up with them. Such patients may be back on the golf course the day after therapy is begun.

Because the response to prednisone is so very striking, some physicians have suggested using less dangerous anti-inflammatory agents such as aspirin or indomethacin for milder cases of polymyalgia rheumatica. In a few instances, such treatment has been successful, but most doctors prefer to treat this condition definitively with prednisone.

No restrictions on activity are required and patients may resume their normal activities after treatment. As the steroid is decreased and eventually discontinued, it is not unusual for some mild symptoms to return, but these usually pose little problem.

If your problem is polymyalgia rheumatica, proceed now to Part II, page 87.

POLYMYOSITIS AND DERMATOMYOSITIS (PM, DM)

Polymyositis and its close relative dermatomyositis are diseases of the muscle and skin that cause not only pain but also weakness and destruction of the muscle. The inflammation (*itis*) in the muscles results in destruction of the muscle fibers.

Along with this process in the muscles, most patients have some involvement of the skin, with skin rash and changes in the skin blood vessels. While the cause of polymyositis is not known, the damage appears to occur because the body's blood cell lymphocytes have become sensitized to the person's own muscle and attack that muscle.

Features

These muscle disorders can occur in any age group and in either sex. In childhood dermatomyositis, the muscle weakness is profound and, after years, the damaged muscles may be permanently replaced by calcium deposits (calcinosus) that can further limit motion.

Because this is predominately a disease of muscles, weakness is the biggest problem. It affects many muscles throughout the body, particularly those of the upper arms, upper legs, and neck region. The involved muscles are weak, frequently tender, and frequently painful. The weakness often is such that the patient cannot get up from a straight chair without assistance and may not be able to lift the head from the bed while lying flat. Problems with the upper swallowing muscles can cause a nasal speech pattern and difficulty in swallowing solid foods. Patients may have trouble climbing stairs or holding their arms out straight to the side.

The skin can be involved. The blood vessels dilate, giving an unusual lavender or heliotrope color to the skin in certain areas. Most frequently, these areas are the eyelids, the knuckles, and the ends of the fingers around the fingernails. A red rash may be seen over much of the rest of the body. There may be some swelling in these regions, but the color changes are most characteristic. Other body organs can be involved; most troublesome is involvement of the lungs. The fingers may be afflicted with Raynaud's phenomenon, in which they turn white and blue in response to cold.

Although the lungs are not often directly involved, they nevertheless constitute the major problem. Weakness in the swallowing muscles or in the breathing muscles can lead to swallowing food "the wrong way" into the lungs or to inability to breathe energetically enough.

Dermatomyositis and polymyositis can be caused by underlying cancer, although this is quite unusual. Practically never is a tumor found in a patient below the age of 40 or 50, and over that age only 10 or 20 percent of the cases are associated with tumors.

In the laboratory, the main clues to the disease are found by tests of muscle enzymes. Two enzymes in particular, the creatine phosphokinase (CPK) together with the aldolase, are usually elevated. (Other enzymes that may be elevated include the SGOT and SGPT.) Other tests are less rewarding; the sedimentation rate may be elevated or not, the blood counts are usually normal, and abnormal antibodies or rheumatoid factors are usually absent. X-rays help very little, since the soft tissues do not show up well on X-ray. An exception is the chest X-ray, which can provide some information about involvement of the lungs. Calcinosis can also be seen on X-ray. Another test, the electromyogram, tests the electrical function of the nerves and muscles. Sometimes this test will help to distinguish polymositis from a disease of the nerves.

Biopsy of the muscle, in which a small piece of a leg muscle or an upper arm muscle is inspected under the microscope, is the definitive test. Inflammation in the muscle is vividly seen under the microscope. Unfortunately, since the disease does not affect every muscle equally, a negative biopsy may merely indicate that a diseased spot was missed. If a weak and tender muscle is biopsied, the result will usually be positive.

Prognosis

This is a serious but variable disease. It is one of the connective-tissue diseases and, as such, is more than just arthritis or rheumatism. In fact, many people would not call it a form of arthritis at all, since the joints are not often involved. Some patients die within five years of the start of the disease; this mortality includes many older patients who have a cancer associated with their disease. On the other hand, many other patients do extremely well. They may respond quickly to treatment, the disease may go away, and, after a period of months, the medicine may be discontinued and they may return to totally normal living. Such cases of polymyositis are "one-shot"—a single episode of illness that lasts some months, then disappears, never to recur. Other patients have a progressive form that can be difficult to treat. This is another extremely variable disease.

The greatest dangers of polymyositis come from involvement of the lungs. Because the muscles in the chest wall are weak, breathing is weak and the patient may not be able to get enough oxygen. Further, since the swallowing mechanism in the throat can be weakened, food may accidently be inhaled into the lungs and cause a serious pneumonia. So, patients without involvement of the lungs or of the swallowing muscles have a better prognosis.

The mainstay of treatment is corticosteroid medication, usually prednisone (p. 108). These powerful drugs are given to almost all patients and usually result in return of the muscle enzymes to normal over several weeks and a gradual increase in muscle strength over the following two to twelve months. Usually the steroids are then tapered to lower doses to decrease toxic reactions. Unfortunately, when steroids are used for long periods of time in high dosages, they cause wasting and weakness of the muscles. There is potential danger that the medicine may contribute to weakness in a disease that already has weakness as its principal problem. Aspirin (p. 98) and other anti-inflammatory drugs are occasionally useful to reduce muscle inflammation.

If the disease is not easily controlled with prednisone or if the prednisone cannot be tapered to less toxic levels, many physicians will add experimental immunosuppressant drugs. These are frequently successful. Most commonly used is methotrexate (p. 125). Azathioprine (Imuran) is another frequently used immunosuppressant agent (p. 125).

There is controversy about how long patients require treatment. Some physicians feel that most patients need to continue treatment for life. In our clinic, approximately half of our patients get off medication within several years. A patient with this disease, however, should expect to be taking medication for some time.

There has also been controversy about the role of exercise in polymyositis. It has been pointed out that exercise will increase the inflammation slightly and will increase the blood levels of the muscle enzymes, which are already abnormally high. On the other hand, exercise preserves the function of the muscles and provides a stimulus to make the muscles stronger. We tell our patients to exercise regularly but gently, gradually increasing the scope of their activities. All of the affected muscles should be worked through their entire range of motion each day to prevent stiffness. Steady exercise to build up strength can consist of walking or swimming or bicycling. We prefer that patients don't overdo exercise until they are conditioned, but that they build slowly toward a stronger exercise program with the goal of restoring normal strength.

It is crucial for the patient to recognize that the process of regaining strength is a very long one. Any time the muscular system is out of condition, the retraining process is lengthy. The body must put many pounds of muscle together and that muscle must become trained and mature. Even without a disease, it may take six to twelve months to regain strength after an enforced period of idleness; with myositis this period may be even longer. The patient should continue to increase activity but should not expect that return of full strength or of a normal muscular appearance will occur over a short period of time.

Smoking, because it injures the lungs, should be discontinued. Patients with Raynaud's phenomenon should keep generally warm and take care of their hands, which will be sensitive to damage from the cold. Patients with trouble swallowing who run the risk of aspiration pneumonia should eat their meals sitting up. They should remain in a sitting or standing position until two or three hours after the last meal of the day, so the stomach has a chance to empty before they lie down. Eating softer foods that pass more easily through the digestive tract may also be helpful.

If your problem is Polymyositis or Dermatomyositis, proceed to Part II, page 87.

Local Conditions:

Injury, Inflammation, and Repair

Detailed discussion of certain other local conditions and their treatment appears in Part III, problems 7 through 17. The following list suggests some of these problems.

- Metatarsalgia—problem 7

- Achilles tendinitis—problem 8

- Heel-spur syndrome—problem 8

- Sprained ankle—problem 9

- Cervical neck strain—problem 13

- Frozen shoulder—problem 14

- Tennis elbow—problem 15

- Carpal-tunnel syndrome—problem 16

BURSITIS

A *bursa* is a small sac of tissue similar to the synovial tissue that lines the joints. The bursa sac contains a lubricating fluid and the bursa is designed to ease the movement of muscle across muscle or of muscle across bone. A bursa does not connect to the joint space of a nearby joint but is a separate sac. Bursae can become inflamed as part of a general inflammation of the synovial tissue, but usually an individual experiences bursitis one or two bursae at a time rather than as part of a major disease process.

"Housemaid's knee" is a popular term for *prepatellar bursitis*, in which the bursa in front and just below the kneecap is inflamed. *Olecranon bursitis* occurs over the point of the elbow, and sometimes a fluid-filled sac may be visible at that point. *Subdeltoid bursitis* occurs in the shoulder—or more precisely, the outer aspect of the upper arm. There are literally dozens of similar bursae in the body and any of them can become inflamed in a particular instance.

Features

Bursitis is inflammation of a bursa and results in localized pain. Sometimes the pain is on both sides of the body, as with both knees. There is pain when the inflamed area is pressed and heat or redness is common. If the bursa is located close enough to the skin, swelling can be seen.

Bursitis comes on relatively suddenly, within hours to days. It frequently follows injury to the area, repeated pressure on the area, or overuse. In the shoulder particularly, it may be associated with tendinitis or calcific tendinitis and can be part of the "frozen shoulder" problem (see problem 14, Part III).

Prognosis

Almost all episodes of bursitis will subside within several days to several weeks, but may recur. If the process causing the bursitis is continued, the bursitis may persist; otherwise, it follows a normal healing course over a period of one week to ten days. Some people seem more prone to bursitis than do others and have recurrent problems throughout their lives. If the affected part is held rigid, some residual stiffness may result; otherwise, no crippling whatsoever should result from bursitis.

Treatment

If the problem is tolerable, treat it with "tincture of time." Wait for the body to control and heal the process. Avoid the precipitating cause if you are able to identify it. Use drugs very sparingly; the process is local and sytemic drugs like aspirin are not very helpful. Resting the part will speed reduction of the inflammation and you may want to use a sling or other device to increase the rest. Gentle warmth provided by a heating pad or warm bath frequently makes the bursitis feel better. The affected area should be worked through its full range of motion several times daily, even if it is a bit tender, to prevent stiffness developing in the part. But remember, patience and avoidance of reinjury are the major tactics.

If the discomfort persists for a number of weeks despite the measures outlined above, see the doctor. The doctor may recommend that you continue the same general measures discussed here. Alternatively, an anti-inflammatory agent may be prescribed; these help a few people, but are generally just a way of buying a little more patience from the patient. Finally, the doctor may inject the bursa with corticosteroids (p. 106). These injections are usually successful and not overly painful. They are relatively free of side effects and most physicians feel they are appropriate treatment for a local condition if it is severe.

For a local problem above, check medication in Chapter 4, page 95, and read about the particular local problem in Part III.

LOW BACK SYNDROMES

Pain in the low back has been called the "curse of the erect posture." From an engineering standpoint, when humans developed a standing posture, the spine developed a double bend, concave in the lower back and convex in the upper back. The back is a complex mechanism with hundreds of ligaments and scores of joints; it is not surprising that injury to this complicated organ occurs in over one-half of all people. Pain can be extremely severe and has been compared with the pain of childbirth, kidney stones, or a heart attack. Low back pain results in as much long-term disability and as many days lost from work as does almost any other illness or injury. Yet, as we will see, it is always difficult to be sure what is going on in any individual case. Further discussion of back pain can be found in Part III, problem 12, "Pain in the Low Back."

The spine consists of a stack of bones, the vertebrae. Each vertebra is connected to the next one by ligaments that cross the vertebral disks. The disks separate the bones much like mushrooms on a shish kebab. Long ligaments run up and down the length of the spine. Muscles attach each vertebra to the ones directly adjacent; other muscles bridge two vertebrae, and three, and four, and so forth. In addition to the disks separating the vertebrae, there are small joints that provide two additional points of contact and movement. These small joints are bridged by ligaments and have synovial tissue within them just like larger joints.

Problems with the disk itself will be discussed in the following section; most low back syndromes, however, are due to problems with one of the back parts mentioned above—the ligaments, the muscles, the joint synovium, or the joint ligaments. Additionally, obese people may have little ruptures of fat through the back tissues and pain from that event.

All minor injuries of the back look and act about the same. A major disk problem, a *herniated nucleus pulposis,* is different and may involve nerve injury. From the outside, neither the doctor nor the patient can tell exactly which tissue was initially injured. Wherever the problem started, a larger portion of the back becomes involved as the body works to immobilize the part to allow its healing. In such cases, muscle spasm and widespread pain is the rule.

Features

Low back syndromes usually result from an injury. The injury is usually obvious, but in at least one-third of patients no incident can be remembered. Muscle spasm provides protection for the injured part by helping to immobilize the back, but this spasm is itself painful. Except for the spasm, which is unique to the back, think of a low back problem as analogous to the more familiar sprain of an ankle. The pain and local swelling are maximum within 24 hours, remain acute and severe for 24 to 72 hours, are somewhat nagging for another week, and require perhaps six weeks to heal back to full strength. Reinjury is very common and starts the timetable all over again. Frequent reinjury can lead to chronic sprains that are more difficult to treat and take a longer time to heal.

The pain is usually most pronounced in the concave portion of the lower back and may frequently radiate to the buttocks. There is pain in the areas of muscle spasm and, on subsequent days, the pain may rise higher in the back as the tired muscles that have been in spasm begin to complain loudly. The pain should not go down into the calf, if it does run down a leg, it is a reason to see the doctor.

The most frequent injury is a sudden hyperextension, in which the lower body continues forward and the upper body is suddenly arched backward. However, all kinds of injuries can result in these syndromes. Injuries occur most frequently in the overweight or inactive individual, or in the individual who exercises only episodically. Good muscle tone and regular exercise protect the back and decrease the risk of these conditions.

Prognosis

About half of patients with low back syndromes have only one to three episodes over a lifetime; the remainder have more episodes than this. Prognosis for the individual episode is excellent and the chances of a serious problem involving pressure on nerves or requiring spinal surgery are less than one percent. If the pain runs down into the legs, particularly the outside of the legs and particularly below the knee, the prognosis is more guarded and greater care in management and in the consideration of surgery is necessary.

If the pain is somewhat less dramatic but lasts for a period of many weeks or months, is worse in the morning, is rather slow in developing, gets better with exercise during the day, and occurs in a person below age 40, ankylosing spondylitis, discussed earlier, should be suspected. Common low back syndromes may loosen up a little bit with activity, but by and large get worse if you overdo before the healing is complete.

Treatment

The injury must heal and this takes time. For the acute painful problem, two possible treatment strategies are acceptable. A third one is not. First, there is the "least pain" way. This involves bed rest, a bed board to provide firm support, sometimes a small pillow beneath the low back if this increases comfort, heat beginning the second day, and pain relievers and muscle relaxants as required to provide comfort.

The second is the "natural" way, in which the patient is up and around as the pain allows, avoids pain relievers, and does not use muscle relaxants.

The third (and unacceptable) way is the "reinjury" way, in which the patient is up and around *and* uses pain relievers and muscle relaxants. The body will heal this problem if left alone. However, if you blunt the pain response of the body and interfere with the immobilization provided naturally by muscle spasm, then reinjury is likely and will delay healing.

You can prevent reinjury by greatly limiting activity—this is the "least pain" way. Or, you can prevent reinjury by allowing the pain reflex and the muscle spasm to protect the injured point—this is the "natural" way. But, if you combine these strategies, you are asking for a long-term problem.

After the acute injury is over, it is time to begin thinking about preventing the next one. Control of weight involves not only reducing to a good body weight but also constant maintenance of that weight. Development of gentle, regular, graded activity to strengthen the spine and improve muscle tone is important. Back protection techniques can help prevent injury when lifting or using the back for different tasks. And specific back exercises can help to strengthen the muscles on the outside of the back and also those that are inside and unseen. By gradually increasing activity, most patients with low back syndromes can return to any activity desired. Even horseback riding and heavy labor are entirely possible if the progression to full activity is patient and gradual. Part III, problem 12, "Pain in the Low Back," discusses these treatment approaches in greater detail.

HERNIATED LUMBAR DISK

Aye, there's the rub. The problem with herniated disks is that they can rub on nerves and cause nerve damage, with serious problems in areas distant from the back. Luckily, few back problems are actually herniated lumbar disks, and even most herniated disks will get better without surgery. Many physicians think that lumbar disks are overdiagnosed and perhaps overtreated. The potential problem is the compression of the nerves, and the following discussion should help you understand this problem.

The stack of vertebrae in the spine are separated by fibrous intervertebral disks, each about one-third inch in height. The outer portion of this disk is fibrous tissue called the *annulus fibrosis* and the center portion is a softer, more gelatinous material called the *nucleus pulposis*. This forms an energy-absorbing yet flexible material that helps cushion the spine while allowing it to move in a supple fashion. Above and below the intervertebral disks are the cartilage end plates of the vertebrae; these are thin layers of cartilage that surface the bones. With increasing age and increasing cumulative injury to the spine, the disk becomes a bit more scarred in the center and a bit narrower. Osteoarthrosis changes can occur next to the disk, with bone spurs growing out from the vertebrae. This process is very slow and usually doesn't cause any symptoms. It does make us get about an inch shorter as we grow older.

A major problem occurs when there is a sudden herniation of the disk. This is a little bit like biting into a chocolate eclair. The gelatinous material in the center of the disk herniates through a tear in weakened fibers and a glob of the interior disk substance is now on the outside of the disk.

This glob would eventually be reabsorbed by normal body mechanisms, leaving a slightly narrower disk space and without symptoms. But the herniated disk material can press on the nerves that go out from the spine, and that's where the rub comes in.

Features

Acute herniated disks tend to occur in the third or fourth decade of life, and less frequently in older individuals. The disk that is most degenerated has become scarred and cannot rupture any longer.

A disk can rupture at any level of the spine, but most frequently one of the bottom two disks is involved. These are the disk between the sacrum and the lowest lumbar vertebra and the disk between the fourth and the fifth lumbar vertebrae, both in the low back. Usually the rupture will occur just to one side of the midline in the back part of the disk. This is an area that is relatively undefended by other ligaments. It can happen on either side, but usually not on both sides at once.

Very rarely, the disk will rupture in the middle and cause immediate severe nerve problems by compressing all of the contents of the spinal canal. Patients with this condition suffer back pain as well as an immediate inability to urinate; in this situation (and this situation alone) immediate surgery is required.

The more classical kind of nerve compression affects just one side and results in *sciatica*, which is irritation of some of the fibers that lead to the sciatic nerve. Depending on how much compression and what level, there may be loss of the reflexes in the leg, numbness of the leg, paralysis or weakness of parts, or total loss of feeling in some areas. Pain is frequently aggravated by a cough or a sneeze, and raising the straightened leg on the affected side increases the pain, often dramatically.

Many patients describe two different kinds of pain. One is a deep, aching pain in the back that runs down the back of the affected buttock and the other is a sharp, needlelike pain that runs down the outside of the leg beyond the knee down the outer part of the calf and into the outer portion of the foot.

The back is frequently in spasm as it is with any back injury, and it will assume a position (curvature of the spine) that relieves the pressure on the nerve root. Thus, the spasm can prevent nerve damage.

Some doctors feel that a number of the minor back problems discussed in the previous section are actually disk protrusions that do not cause nerve pressure. This may well be true, but there is no reason to consider a disk a more serious problem unless some symptoms of rubbing on the nerve roots are present.

Prognosis

Surgery is recommended for between 5 and 30 percent of patients with nerve-root compression, this figure depending partly on the particular doctor consulted. We feel that the lower figures are more appropriate and that back surgery should be carefully considered, preferably with two or more physicians' opinions, before the final surgical decision. As is well known, even after back surgery the problem may recur, if not at the disk that was removed, then at another level. Further, the back surgery itself disrupts at least a part of this very complex organ and can result in some scarring and stiffness.

On the other hand, most people with disk problems recover without surgery and most are able to return to work and eventually to full activity. The time required may be discouragingly long and extend over many weeks or months, but the motivated and careful patient will usually achieve good results without surgery.

Treatment

Bed rest, in the position of greatest comfort is central to most treatment. Some doctors recommend a pillow under the knees or under the low back, others emphasize a straight, firm bed board. The key is the position of greatest comfort. Pain medications may be required, but, as emphasized in the previous section, they should not be used to allow activity that would otherwise be impossible, since this may encourage more nerve damage and slower healing.

Manipulation is employed by some doctors and other practitioners. Several maneuvers are used, including straight leg raising on the affected side, bending the knees back to the chest and pushing on them with a circular motion, and backward stretching. These procedures sometimes work—with a little pop, the symptoms go away. Presumably what happens is that the herniated material shifts position slightly, relieving the pressure on the nerve. Unfortunately, the potential exists for completely breaking the nerve root by these maneuvers and we recommend that they be undertaken only by an experienced individual. All patients with symptoms of nerve root compression should be under a doctor's care.

Hospital bed rest may be required in a few cases. Some physicians use traction, but others argue strongly against it. Some physicians employ a corset to help support the spine; we have not had a great deal of success with corsets.

Surgery is required for patients with urine retention or major nerve syndromes. The surgery is usually successful in relieving the immediate nerve pressure, but problems can recur and back pain may persist.

In the asymptomatic interval following healing of an acute disk injury, exercises to strengthen the paraspinal muscles are helpful and carefully graded return to activity is important.

If you have a back problem, check any drugs required in Chapter 4, then proceed to Problem 12, Part III.

General Conditions:

Aching All Over

A whole host of disease conditions have been termed *nonarticular rheumatism,* a most unfortunate and confusing term. Alternate terms—fibrositis, psychogenic rheumatism, osteoporosis, psycho-physiological musculoskeletal reaction, anxiety neurosis, depressive reaction—are just as confusing. None of these terms is particularly accurate, and none of them can be applied to all patients with symptoms of long-term general aching and the total absence of evidence for an actual disease process. The patient is confused—in part because the doctor is likely to be confused as well. There are no really clear distinctions in this disease area.

The discussion in this chapter falls under three headings: fibrositis, psychogenic rheumatism, and depression and arthritis. These distinctions are not clear and you may want to read each section carefully to see which aspects of the discussion seem to apply to you.

Part of the frustration of these syndromes is that they are nonobjective. That is, nothing in the physical examination or in the laboratory examination suggests that anything at all is wrong with the patient. Further, nothing really happens to the patient as time goes on. The symptoms may go away or stay, but they don't get worse. Over a period of time most symptoms disappear. Recent research has given us some insights into the condition long called fibrositis; this condition is now developing some of the characteristics of an understandable disease. Nevertheless, none of the theories about these conditions is totally convincing; none should obscure the fact that basically these are minor problems that, with time, generally get better.

FIBROSITIS

Fibrositis is one of the terms used for aching all over. Recently, it has been defined more precisely in terms of three distinguishing characteristics:

77

aching in many parts of the body, an abnormal sleep pattern that results in marked morning stiffness and fatigue, and local tenderness in many of fourteen specific places. The last two features are quite new and are interesting to us because of their similarity to the "muscle-contraction" theory that has been the basis of our approach to these conditions.

The muscle-contraction theory holds that there is tone in a normal resting muscle that exerts a certain amount of force on the tendons at either end of the muscle. When a patient has abnormally high muscle-contraction tone, or fails to relax the muscle at night when asleep, the abnormal pull on the tendons can cause inflammation and pain. This phenomenon is related to tension and to the so-called tension headache, which causes tenderness at the base of the skull where the neck muscles attach. Tension headaches are believed to result from excessive tension in the neck musculature. Fibrositis is similar to tension headache, but it affects many parts of the body.

Features

The "tender points" are particular body locations that are normally somewhat tender; most readers can identify these points on their own bodies. Firm pressure applied to these areas will hurt anyone, but the patient with fibrositis experiences even more pain when these areas are pressed. For example, about halfway between the neck and the shoulder, one can feel the upper border of the trapezius muscle. At midpoint of this muscle there is a tender site. The "tennis elbow" site is just about an inch down the forearm from the outer bump on the side of the elbow when the palm is turned up. This tender spot may feel like a cord. There is also tenderness at the second costochondral junction, next to the breastbone on either side and about an inch or two below the collarbone. A fourth site is in the fat pad on the inside portion of the knee.

The second newly identified characteristic of fibrositis is sleep disturbance. Technically, this is a decrease in *slow wave activity*, the kind of sleep most restful to the muscles. Patients with fibrositis have a very jerky sleep tracing on an electroencephalogram (EEG) when compared with normal people. This sleep pattern is similar to that obtained when healthy persons are kept without sleep for two or three nights. These patterns do not appear in subjects who are thoroughly physically fit, even after sleep deprivation.

So, a pattern of the typical fibrositis patient emerges. There may be an underlying tension problem. The patient is apt to exercise irregularly or inadequately. The sleep disturance, perhaps caused initially by the tension, leads to a state of long-term sleep loss, and the muscles don't have enough rest time during the night. The rest of the syndrome follows more or less from these points.

Prognosis

Medically, these syndromes are benign and carry an excellent prognosis. There will be no crippling and no severe disability. On the other hand, without treatment, the misery may last for many months or years.

Treatment

The principles above suggest a rational treatment program. Exercise, slowly increased and toward full aerobic cardiovascular conditioning and physical tiredness is the most important daily component. Warm baths may be helpful, and a glass of wine in the evening has proved relaxing to some.

Drug treatment is more controversial, since it treats only a symptom and not a cause. Moreover, the quality of the sleep is not improved just by taking a lot of sleeping pills. Most sleeping pills do not counteract this particular kind of sleep disturbance at all and some may actually make it worse. A drug felt useful by some physicians is chlorpromazine (Thorazine), but evidence for its usefulness is not very well established. We use exercise as practically our only therapeutic modality. When a patient is able to walk extensively and to swim, hike, or bicycle regularly, we have seen gradual resolution of the syndrome after a few weeks to a few months. Getting rid of these bothersome symptoms depends on the patient.

PSYCHOGENIC RHEUMATISM

There is a sense in which we all have pain all of the time. The pain fibers linking the body to the brain are continually firing off impulses about some sensation or another. Usually, we suppress and ignore these signals if they are too minor to merit attention. But if we sit quietly and scan our bodies carefully for any painful signals, we can find some at any given moment.

Some people complain of "aching all over." On closer examination, it appears that while their painful sensations are not abnormal, their reaction to these sensations is. These normal sensations have become a medical problem. This is one explanation for psychogenic rheumatism, a very inadequately defined condition.

A frequent common denominator to these painful syndromes is accident litigation, disability-insurance application, or the use of a painful symptom to manipulate another individual. This common denominator is called secondary gain. Pain, a normally undesirable feature, assumes value because it helps in getting someone else to do what the individual wants. Rather than our normal tendency to ignore minor pain impulses, there is an incentive to amplify these sensations and pay attention to them. The patient is very seldom aware of what is happening.

Features

These syndromes can take several forms. The pain can be all over the body or it can be localized in the area of a previous injury, often the neck (whiplash) or the low back (job-related injury). Often, patients report pains that do not follow normal anatomic patterns—that is, they don't follow the course of actual nerves.

Patients are often tense, sometimes angry. The syndromes may merge with fibrositis and the muscle-contraction syndrome.

Laboratory tests and X-rays are normal or, if abnormal, do not explain the symptoms. The symptoms do not respond well to medications or to injections.

Prognosis

Serious problems with the musculoskeletal system are not possible, since this really is not a disease of the musculoskeletal system. The syndrome can be an unhappy one, however, and may persist for months or years. Drug dependency can result and problems with excessive drug use or excessive surgery are the most unfortunate results encountered.

Treatment

Crippling or major disability will not result. Sometimes laboratory tests are ordered by the doctor in an effort to reassure the patient. It is important to honestly identify and to remove any secondary-gain considerations. This syndrome notoriously improves as soon as a lawsuit is settled, whatever the outcome. It may respond to better, more direct communication between a manipulated person and the manipulator. Finally, avoidance of drugs is central to good therapy. Medication is not helpful and offers potential for dependency. Further, the mood-altering effects of commonly prescribed drugs make coping with this frustrating syndrome more difficult.

DEPRESSION AND ARTHRITIS

While we all get depressed sometimes, serious psychiatric depressions constitute major illness. The patient feels helpless and worthless. Everything is down, down, down. Sleep may be disturbed by obsessive, recurring, pessimistic thoughts, and the musculoskeletal system works very slowly. Speech is slow, body movements are slow, and there is frequently stiffness throughout much of the body. These pains and stiffness may be called "rheumatism" or "arthritis"; they are most frequent in older individuals.

Depressive reactions may follow loss of a loved one. These grief reactions, while similar, are ultimately less serious since they resolve after several months of adjustment.

Features

This syndrome is a vague one. It may blend with psychogenic rheumatism or with fibrositis. The sleep-deprivation mechanism that appears to operate in fibrositis probably accentuates the symptoms associated with depression. And the patient may use the musculoskeletal symptoms to explain why he or she just isn't getting along very well, thus using a mechanism of secondary gain like that of psychogenic rheumatism.

Again, the symptoms frequently don't come from specific body areas or follow usual nerve or muscle paths. The depression is general, so these syndromes will involve many parts of the body.

Similar symptoms occur with an inactive thyroid gland. Parkinson's disease, due to hardening of the arteries, is common in the same age group and can result in slowness and stiffness. Both thyroid disease and Parkinson's disease can be well treated, so it is important to recognize their presence.

Prognosis

Again, this is predominantly not a musculoskeletal condition. The prognosis is that of the depressive reaction. In a grief reaction, there is usually a return to normal after four to six months. With severe psychiatric depression, the period may be much longer.

Treatment

These syndromes are a signal to consider major life-style changes, even if the person's age is advanced. It is important to look forward to future events rather than only backward at what has gone before. New activities, new social groups, and new friends should be encouraged. It is a time for physical activity and for staying out of the house, even if such activities must be forced. Plant some young new trees and plan to attend the grand-children's college graduation, even if they are only seven.

Medication may be required for treatment of the depression; such medication is often successful. On the other hand, musculoskeletal drugs should not be used. In particular, drugs like Valium and codeine should be avoided. These drugs are themselves depressants, can aggravate these kinds of symptoms, and may perpetuate the problem. Minor pain-killing medications, such as acetaminophen (Tylenol) may be used, but are unlikely to help a great deal. For further discussion, see Part III, problem 5.

If your problem is a general condition, proceed to Part II, page 87.

The Connective-Tissue Diseases:

Not Quite Arthritis

Five diseases (systemic lupus erythematosus, rheumatoid arthritis, polymyositis, scleroderma, and polyarteritis) are frequently considered cousins of one another and are grouped under the name *connective tissue* diseases. These diseases are also sometimes called *autoimmune* diseases or *collagen-vascular* diseases. We have discussed three of these diseases (lupus, rheumatoid arthritis, and polymyositis) before. They can affect the joints or muscles, and the musculoskeletal part of the disease may be the major manifestation. But these conditions also affect other parts of the body. They involve several of the body organs. Arthritis is part of the picture, and a specialist in arthritis (rheumatologist) is often required for care or consultation.

LUPUS (SLE): A RECAP

Lupus is a disease of autoantibodies. The body's immune system seems to be producing too many antibodies and some of these antibodies attack the tissues of the patient. The joints are one such tissue, but there are many others. Lupus is discussed in Chapter 2, beginning on page 25.

RHEUMATOID ARTHRITIS (RA): A RECAP

Rheumatoid arthritis is listed here to indicate again that it is a systemic disease that affects many parts of the body. RA is discussed in Chapter 2, beginning on page 17.

These diseases of inflamed muscle can affect other parts of the body. They are discussed in Chapter 7, beginning on page 63.

SCLERODERMA

Scleroderma literally means "hard skin." The skin of a scleroderma patient, particularly over the fingers, arms, and sometimes face, can become stiff and bound down. The condition is due to a problem with the circulation through the small blood vessels, which eventually leads to scarring of the skin. If the skin becomes bound down and tight, the hands may become stiff. Because of the circulation problems, ulcers may develop on the fingertips.

Scleroderma, then, is not really arthritis. The problem is in the blood vessels and the skin and tissue around the joints, but it can lead to deformities not unlike those of true arthritis. Actually, when you look at the scleroderma joint tissues under the microscope, some signs of a true arthritis do appear.

The cause of scleroderma is not known. Current research suggests that problems in the smaller blood vessels result in damage to tissues. Earlier theories of too much scar tissue in the body are slowly being discarded, as are theories that antibodies, as in lupus, cause the disease.

Features

Scleroderma patients usually have Raynaud's phenomenon. This phenomenon is a color change of the fingers, usually from white to blue to red, after exposure to cold. Most people with Raynaud's phenomenon do not develop scleroderma, but a few do, and this can be the first sign of scleroderma. *Acrosclerosis* is a medical term referring to hardening of the skin of the fingers and sometimes the toes. This occurs in most patients with scleroderma; sometimes there are calcium deposits beneath the skin as well. Hardening of the skin elsewhere is usually less impressive, but may limit the ability to open the mouth or cause some wrinkling around the eyes and mouth.

The scleroderma process can involve organs other than the skin. Most frequently, the gastrointestinal tract is involved. The esophagus (gullet) can develop changes similar to those of the skin and the swallowing wave can be interrupted. The stomach may become dilated, the small bowel dilated, and outpouchings of a special sort may develop in the colon. Scarring of the lower lungs may occur and, in a few patients, the kidneys become abruptly involved with high blood pressure and kidney failure.

Laboratory findings are not much help in diagnosis. X-rays may show calcium deposits in various places or may reveal the gastrointestinal-tract problems noted above.

Prognosis

Progressive systemic sclerosis (scleroderma) is not progressive, not systemic, and not sclerosis. As with many of the diseases in this section, the name is misleading and unnecessarily ominous. Most patients do not have progressive courses. The disease will be active for a period of perhaps two years and then stabilize or even get better over the following years. It is not systemic in that only certain parts of the body are characteristically affected by scleroderma. Even these are not constant from patient to patient. Many patients have essentially just a mild skin condition. It is not sclerosis (which means "scarring") because scarring is only the accidental result of a problem of inadequate blood supply. The basic problem is inadequate flow through the small blood vessels.

The scleroderma patient frequently worries about the disease progressing to "mummylike" skin or, as it was once put, being "encased in a slowly shrinking, ever contracting, skin of steel." Fortunately, this doesn't happen. The skin involvement with scleroderma remains localized to the fingers, forearms, face, and neck in the overwhelming majority of patients, with perhaps some minor involvement of the toes and lower legs. With the exception of difficulty moving affected finger areas in advanced cases, scleroderma does not usually hamper a normal life-style.

Most people regard the appearance of calcium deposits as a bad sign. In fact, patients with calcinosis do better than other patients with scleroderma. In particular, patients with a syndrome of calcium deposits, Raynaud's phenomenon, esophageal swallowing problems, scleroderma involvement of the fingers, and little red spots called *telangiectasia* do particularly well. These patients are said to have the "CREST" syndrome and they typically lead entirely normal lives.

Somewhere between 5 and 10 percent of patients with scleroderma develop a kidney problem. This is a serious medical complication and can lead to death over a short time. In recent years, medical treatment has been developed and kidney dialysis and transplantation have been useful. The sudden development of high blood pressure or of protein in the urine, a seizure, or decreased vision are worrisome signs in this disease, just as the presence of calcium beneath the skin is a good sign.

Treatment

The patient is the most important factor in successful adjustment to and recovery from this disease. For treatment of complications, however, the physician's role is crucial. It is essential that the patient's attitude toward life and the disease be positive. Good expectations work to increase blood flow through compromised blood vessels. The patient must actively exercise affected areas so as to stretch the skin and preserve full motion of the joints. Exercises such as placing the hand flat on a table and pressing until the fingers are straight, making a fist and then cocking the wrist to stretch the joint further, and so forth, should be repeated several times daily to improve circulation and maintain motion.

Life-style should be as normal as possible. If symptoms of heartburn or stomach upset occur, antacids are appropriate and the doctor should be consulted about treatment for *reflux esophagitis.* Early treatment of heartburn can prevent some later complications. Since the blood flow to the hands is less than perfect, good hand care is important. A cut on the fingers or fingertips may heal more slowly than in a person without the condition. Measures to keep the body warm to minimize Raynaud's phenomenon should include gloves as well as warmth for the trunk and neck areas that control the reflexes for blood flow to the fingers.

When complications occur, corticosteroid medications may be required for inflammation of the muscles. Medicines may be needed for high blood pressure and kidney disease. Antibiotics are successful for some of the gastrointestinal syndromes. Physician care and these powerful medicines can frequently help, but the day-to-day management of the uncomplicated disease depends on the patient.

If your problem is Scleroderma, proceed now to Part II, page 87.

POLYARTERITIS

"Inflammation of many arteries" is the problem with polyarteritis and the very meaning of the word. The arteries that supply blood to the body normally consist of an inner coat, a muscular middle layer, and an outer coat. Inflammation and destruction of all layers of these blood vessels occurs with polyarteritis. The organ for which the blood was sent does not receive the blood and tissue damage occurs.

Several other diseases cause inflammation of the arteries, including polymyalgia rheumatica, described in Chapter 7. The polyarteritis type of blood-vessel inflammation, however, was the first discovered and is probably the most serious.

In recent years scientists have found the cause of some forms of polyarteritis. For example, the hepatitis virus can stimulate the body to form antibodies against the virus; the virus and the antibodies can then combine in the blood and lodge in the blood vessels. These *immune complexes* cause the inflammation that, in turn, causes damage to the vessel. In this case, polyarteritis is caused by a virus.

The key to understanding this complicated disease is its spotty involvement around the body. Various symptoms can be observed in various locations. But each problem has to result from inadequate blood supply caused by an attack on a particular blood vessel.

Features

The lesions of polyarteritis are typically scattered. In the skin they may consist of small spots with a central sore not much bigger than the head of a pin. The skin spot itself may be one-quarter to one-half inch in diameter. These sores may come in "crops"; each sore represents the interruption of blood flow through one small artery. In the lungs, X-rays can show pneumonias or even cavities within the lung that are the result of problems with the blood vessels. When the blood vessel that supplies a nerve is affected, the nerve ceases to work. There may be numbness or inability to use one particular muscle group. For example, there may be a *foot drop*, in which the toes cannot be lifted upward and the foot slaps as the patient walks along. Involvement of the arteries can lead to kidney failure through inflammation of the blood vessels that supply blood to the kidney tissue.

In the laboratory there is little to assist in the diagnosis of polyarteritis. Often the fibrinogen level will be raised; this protein is part of the repair process for blood vessels. The platelet count may also be slightly raised and the sedimentation rate may be elevated.

Plain X-rays show little. In a difficult diagnostic case, an X-ray performed by injecting dye into the blood vessels of the abdomen may show little balloonlike aneurysms of the arteries.

A biopsy is the major technique for establishing a diagnosis of polyarteritis and is almost always required. A biopsy may be of the muscle, of the skin, or of other areas. The pathologist, looking at the biopsy under the microscope, can see the inflammation of the arteries and can establish the diagnosis.

Prognosis

Until recently, the prognosis for polyarteritis has not been good. With current treatment, however, the prognosis is much better. Most patients return to a normal life after a sickness lasting some months, but many have to continue on medication with undesirable side effects for several years. Even now, despite excellent treatment, a few people die after only a few months of disease. Most of the time polyarteritis responds to treatment, but sometimes nothing seems to work.

Treatment

Prednisone (p. 108) is the major medication used and is given in high doses, with all of the resulting side effects. Cytotoxic or immunosuppressive drugs such as Imuran (p. 125) or Cytoxan (p. 124) are frequently used along with the prednisone and have decreased the rate of mortality from the disease. In a disease related to polyarteritis (Wegener's granulomatosis), treatment with both prednisone and an immunosuppressant agent is essential for a good result. Medications are tapered to lower doses over a period of several months to several years and are eventually discontinued in most patients.

PART

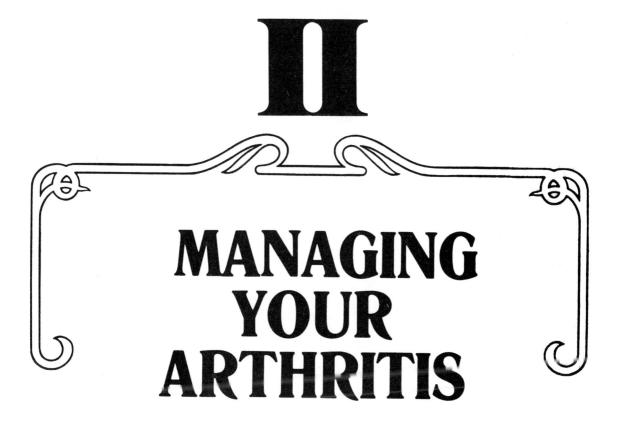

MANAGING YOUR ARTHRITIS

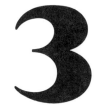

Treatment Begins at Home

YOUR LIFE-STYLE

Your life-style with arthritis should be guided by common sense. There are three major factors that you may be neglecting. Let's consider these first and then proceed to some general conclusions.

Defense against Arthritis

First, consider the defense mechanisms of the body; they are many and wonderful. The body reacts to anything that disturbs its health by means of these mechanisms. In our society we often forget just how useful they are. The cough that clears foreign material or bacteria from our lungs, the diarrhea that helps carry the food toxin outside of our body, the runny nose that takes the virus outside where it can do no harm—all are essential to the maintenance of good health. Yet, curiously, we often consider defense mechanisms to be diseases.

An important defense mechanism is pain. Pain can tell you that you are overusing an injured joint or are interfering with the natural healing of a sprained ligament. Animals do very well with arthritis and muscle problems because they let that internal doctor—pain—guide their activities.

If your pain improves with exercise, then gentle increase in an exercise program makes sense. If pain gets worse or occurs after exercise, that's a signal for backing off from that particular activity. Pain isn't pleasant. You don't need to like it. But it will help you. Don't blunt the pain sensation with pain medications if at all possible. You need the advice given by this unpleasant sensation.

Another defense mechanism is the symptom of fatigue. Fatigue is the body's way of telling you that it needs rest, and you ought to listen to this "doctor" as well. Pain and fatigue provide you with a constant stream of advice about what you should be doing.

Exercise

Second, consider the benefits and drawbacks of exercise. The bones react to exercise and to weight bearing by growing stronger. The body absorbs more calcium, deposits it in the bones, and creates thicker and sturdier support structures. Exercise builds the muscles and increases muscle tone. This creates support across the joints and helps to stabilize the joint. The tendons, as well as the ligaments, gain strength when they are used. Each of these tissues gets weaker when it is not used.

The cartilage of the joint is a most interesting tissue. This gristle does not have a blood supply. It gets oxygen and nourishment and gets rid of waste products by compression—fluid is squeezed into the joint space, then removed and replenished. The health of the cartilage depends on motion, because without motion there is no nourishment of the cartilage. Even a few weeks in a plaster cast may result in cartilage degeneration. In contrast, marathon runners and others who subject their cartilage to great stress throughout life tend not to have excessive degeneration of the cartilage.

Exercise also gives major psychological benefits. It is an excellent way to fight anxiety and depression. The physical tiredness induced by exercise increases the depth of the sleep period, which in turn improves energy and vigor the following day. Further, the social interactions encouraged by exercise are themselves very healthy.

There is one drawback to exercising with arthritis. If the arthritis is an inflammatory synovitis (such as rheumatoid arthritis), exercise of the inflamed part will make the inflammation temporarily worse. For this reason, there is some controversy among doctors about the proper role of rest and exercise. The consensus is that exercise is necessary for all patients with all forms of arthritis. With active synovitis, exercise should be limited (while the active inflammation persists) to levels that do not greatly increase the pain and inflammation.

Rest does just the opposite of exercise. It reduces inflammation if such is present. It increases calcium loss from bone, allows the muscles and tendons to weaken, and fails to nourish the cartilage. It has the psychological disadvantage of encouraging dependency.

To Meet the Challenge

Third, consider what you want to accomplish. Life-style is your own choice. But the clock is ticking. You would like to increase the days of full function in your life. If you put off the challenge posed by your arthritis to "when you feel better," you may never get around to it. Or, when you finally do decide to start a program of active living, your muscles, bones, tendons and habits may be so out of shape that getting back into condition for normal activity will be a long-term process. When you consider what you want to accomplish, you may find that some adjustments are realistically necessary. For the most part, however, you can do whatever you set out to do.

Now, a caution about doctors. We can't always tell how much you hurt. We have trouble telling exactly how tired and fatigued you are. We tend to give you arbitrary rules, good for most people but perhaps not quite right for you. Studies show that you don't take our advice about activity and life-style very seriously anyhow. So, these decisions are largely up to you and your common sense. Let's test the principles above on some of the questions most commonly asked.

SHOULD I WORK?

Sure, if you can. Some physical occupations may need adjustment because they put too much stress across joints and increase pain and discomfort. Or, if your arthritis is severe, you may be incapable of doing them. But there is usually an alternate job or better job that you can do very well. You may have to make some adjustments at home. If you work, you may have to simplify your home life in one way or another. A smaller house, domestic help, or whatever. The payoffs for working are satisfaction, productivity, pride, and money. And if you don't blunt your pain response with too much pain medication, it's difficult to hurt yourself or injure your joints, because the arthritis process itself will prevent that.

HOW MUCH EXERCISE?

Work up to it. Listen for the pain message. Go slow. The principles of conditioning are well understood by coaches and by good athletes. They consist of regular exercise, slowly increased to the desired level. Some setbacks are to be expected during an exercise program. Don't let them scare you off. They are not permanent. Keep at it.

WHAT KIND OF EXERCISE?

There are two major kinds of exercise and, depending on your problems, you will want to mix them in differing degrees; more specific discussions appear in Part III. First, exercise as an activity, gently graded, builds muscle and heart tone, strengthens ligaments, decreases anxiety, and does a lot of other good things. Second, therapeutic exercises directed at problems with specific areas of the body can increase the motion at joints or strengthen specific regions, such as the upper leg muscles.

Here there are three "do's" and a "don't." *Do* be regular and slowly progressive with your exercise program. *Do* stretching and range-of-motion exercises on a regular basis. Affected joints should be stretched to the limits of discomfort several times daily in order to prevent permanent stiffness at the joints. *Do* smooth regular exercises with many repetitions. Examples of such exercises are swimming, bicycling, and walking. No tremendously strenuous actions are required by these exercises. They can be gradually increased and, if you have to stop at some point, there's no particular social pressure.

Don't do high-tension exercises requiring forces across the joints. Weight lifting, ball squeezing, and so forth place more stress across the injured joint than the joint needs. Intermediate are such sports as tennis, bowling, and golf, which require strength and jerky movements to varying degrees. Bicycling puts stress across the knee and should be done with care if the knees are sore or swollen.

WHEN SHOULD I REST?

When you are tired. The dilemma of rest versus exercise causes much misunderstanding. Doctors usually recommend both rest and exercise, and patients perceive this as a contradiction. Actually, the two modes should alternate. When you are tired listen to the fatigue message coming from your body. If you require a nap midday or a nap after work, then take it. Try to keep the rest periods relatively short and don't be too afraid to get a little bit tired. Naps during the day may take away from your night sleep. By doing too much napping during the day, you can get into a vicious cycle that has you feeling tired all of the time.

WHAT ABOUT DIET?

Diet and arthritis: this curious theme repeats itself in dozens of quack remedies. Every patient with arthritis, at some point, wonders if the disease is the result of some improper eating habit or if the disease would disappear if correct foods were eaten. The central question, "Why did I get arthritis?" seldom has a good answer, so we tend to accept any answer at all.

Quacks have suggested that fish diets, oils, vitamins, mineral supplements, vegetarian diets, honey and vinegar, fresh fruits and laxatives, low fat, high fat, low protein, high protein, and every other imaginable combination of foods will cure arthritis. Each diet contradicts the others.

There is no special diet for arthritis. The only known relationship between food and arthritis is with gout, where a diet heavy in purines will increase the chances of an attack. Patients with gout should avoid sweetbreads, liver, kidney, and brain, since these foods are very rich in purines.

If you think about it, you know that diet is not the answer. You didn't eat any differently than anyone else before you had your arthritis. You also know that there are many kinds of arthritis and that there cannot be a single cause or cure for all kinds. It is tempting to accept a simple answer to a complicated problem, but it just isn't that easy. Keep your common sense active.

Weight control is important for the prevention and the treatment of many kinds of arthritis and, in this sense, diet is very important. In Part III, problem 6, the subject of obesity is discussed.

A balanced, moderate diet is part of the good health habits you want to develop. The body needs raw materials of various sorts for daily work and for repair. Foods from each of the major groups, vitamins, minerals, and fluid are all required—but not in excess. The diet good for your general health is good for your arthritis. Enjoy.

WHAT ABOUT CLIMATE?

Some people with arthritis can forecast the weather. An approaching low-pressure system, with a falling barometer, causes an increase in pain and stiffness in such patients. Scientists have tested this phenomenon in pressure chambers and it is indeed true.

So, should you move to Arizona? The warmth of the desert sun might bake out some of those aches and the high-pressure weather systems over the desert will minimize the pains caused by changing barometric pressure.

The answer: Sometimes. The course of arthritis is not changed by living in desert areas. Comfort is improved for some patients and not for others. Is slight improvement in comfort worth the disruption entailed by a move to a new place? Often not. If you are thinking seriously about such a move, take an extended vacation to the new place first. If you are going to feel better on the desert, improvement will be evident within a few weeks. If the combination of vacation and sun doesn't help very much, a permanent move is not a good idea.

EXPECTATIONS

Your expectations are the key to how well you will do with your arthritis. Roosevelt declared during the Depression that "the only thing we have to fear is fear itself." Although with overuse this phrase has become dated, for the patient with arthritis, nothing is truer.

Expectations for individual patients vary. Realistic expectations, however, are almost always good. The patient who assumes the worst is in big trouble. Such patients often get into a cycle much like the following: a job is given up because of anticipated future disability, the patient takes a dependent role at home, self-image is decreased and personal pride diminished. The patient uses the disease to manipulate others, friends are lost, the patient never leaves home so no new friends are made, and a downward spiral into passive isolation and unhappiness continues.

A handicap, if you have one from arthritis, is just that. It is just a handicap. Eyeglasses, a hearing aid, a wooden leg, a crutch. Arthritis, heart disease, cancer, stroke. There are two kinds of people: those who have a handicap now and those who are going to have one.

Illness is a human experience. Many patients become finer persons because of the insights, the sensitivity, and the empathy induced by living with a chronic illness. The ability to understand others, to offer hope and help, and to serve as a model for those around you may be enhanced by the presence of arthritis.

It is not easy to see any positive side to a disability and to escape depression and anger. In the first months of a long disease it may be impossible. If your arthritis is serious, it may represent the greatest challenge of your life. Meeting the challenge can be your greatest satisfaction. Christiaan Barnard performed the first heart-transplant operation and innumerable cardiac surgical procedures—*with* rheumatoid arthritis. Rosalind Russell maintained a vigorous public life of tremendous public service while battling severe rheumatoid arthritis. Jerry Walsh retired from professional baseball because of rheumatoid arthritis and spent an energetic life crusading against quack treatments and for sound management of arthritis. The list goes on.

Think forward. Make plans. Set goals. Carry them out. You need a bit more will and determination and self-discipline than others. But the future is still yours.

4

The Drug Scene:
What Medications Help Arthritis?

Probably you don't know nearly enough about this subject. If the truth be told, your doctor is tired of repeating the same information to person after person, over and over. No drug is simple, and full explanation inevitably takes a lot of time. Unfortunately, this time is not often available.

And you forget, too. The interview with your doctor is an intensive expe rience. All too frequently discussion of the prescribed treatment serves as a quick end to the encounter—too little time for such an important subject. In this chapter, the discussions you have been having with your physician are repeated. Read the ones you need. Reread if you forget.

DRUGS TO REDUCE INFLAMMATION

The most important arthritis medicines reduce inflammation. Inflammation is part of the normal healing process. The body increases blood flow and mobilizes imflammatory cells to repair wounded tissues or to eliminate bacterial invaders. The inflammation causes the area to be warm, red, tender, and often swollen. It is important to recognize that inflammation can be a normal process in order to understand the potential problems of drugs that reduce inflammation.

In four categories of arthritis (synovitis, attachment arthritis, crystal arthritis, and muscle inflammation), the inflammation causes damage and thus suppression of the inflammation can be helpful in treatment. In other categories (cartilage degeneration, infection, local conditions, and general conditions), there is little inflammation or the inflammation may be necessary for the healing process. So, you don't always want an anti-inflammatory drug just because you have arthritis. In four categories—yes; in four other categories—often no.

Aspirin is the most important single drug for arthritis. Not only is it useful itself, it serves as a model for understanding the benefits and problems of medical treatment of arthritis.

Aspirin is the most important drug in the world and the most misunderstood. It is sold by the carload and it causes more total side effects than any other drug, yet it is among the safest drugs currently used in the United States. Its very familiarity has led to its loss of stature. Sometimes, it is equated with physician neglect, as in "Take two aspirin and call me in the morning." Yet it is said to be so powerful that the Food and Drug Administration, if presented with aspirin as a new drug, today would not license it. The scare press delights in reporting the hazards of aspirin—bleeding from the stomach or liver damage. The same press reports the next day that aspirin may prevent heart attacks by thinning the blood. These contradictions dominate our daily encounters with aspirin.

If used properly, aspirin is a marvelous drug for many kinds of arthritis. If not used correctly, it can lead to real frustration. Read the next several paragraphs carefully; they suggest what you need to know about aspirin specifically, but also illustrate general principles you need to know about all arthritis medications.

You must know the difference between the terms *analgesic* and *anti-inflammatory*. *Analgesic* means "pain killing." *Anti-inflammatory* means that the redness and swelling are reduced. Aspirin provides minor pain relief and is helpful for headaches, sunburn, or other familiar problems. But it can also be a major anti-inflammatory agent and can actually decrease the swelling and tissue damage in arthritis. Taken correctly, it is as powerful as moderate doses of cortisone.

The dosage is the difference. The pain-killing effects of aspirin are maximal after two tablets (10 grains). If you take more aspirin, you don't really get any more pain relief. You can repeat this analgesic (pain-killing) dose every four hours because it tends to wear off in about that time. In contrast, the anti-inflammatory activity requires high and sustained blood levels of the aspirin. A patient must take 12 to 24 tablets (5 grains each) each day and the process must be continued for weeks to obtain the full effect.

This distinction is critically important. The pain-killing activity of aspirin is not effective for major forms of arthritis. The anti-inflammatory activity is the desired effect. But this requires that the treatment be undertaken seriously, with medical supervision, and be maintained for a prolonged period. Since the effective doses are so high, most patients will encounter some side reactions and the dosage level will require adjustment. This takes us to a second consideration.

You must know the difference between allergy and side effects. Patients often maintain that they can't tolerate a drug because of problems they had with it a while back. When the doctor asks what drugs you are allergic to, you may mention such drugs because of the problems you experienced. Most of the time, these problems are related to a side effect of the drug, not an allergy.

Allergy is relatively rare; side effects are common. Only a few people get an allergy, but everyone experiences side effects if they are given enough of a drug. There are different symptoms. A skin rash, wheezing in the lungs, or a runny nose generally mean allergy. Nausea, abdominal pain, ringing in the ears, and headache usually mean side effects. If you have an allergy to a drug, that is a good reason to avoid that drug in the future. If you have side effects to a drug, usually it means that you need one or another trick to get your body to tolerate the drug better or perhaps just a little lower dose.

These considerations are particularly important with aspirin. The treatment range is just below the level that gives side effects. So, most patients receiving aspirin for anti-inflammatory purposes will have some ringing in the ears or some nausea. This is just a reason to slow down a little bit and to establish what dose is the exactly correct one for you. If you don't know this principle, you are going to give up too soon on a superb drug and you won't get better. Your knowledge is critical to your health.

You must know about drug absorption and drug interactions. Food delays the absorption of a medicine into your body. With some drugs the presence of food in your stomach will actually prevent the absorption of the medication. But food also protects the stomach lining and can make taking a drug more comfortable. Thus, although food may decrease the effectiveness of a medication, it also may decrease certain side effects by protecting the stomach. By and large, antacids (Maalox, Mylantin, Gelusil) act just about the same as food; they delay absorption but protect the stomach.

Some medications are coated to protect the stomach; the coating is designed to dissolve after the tablet has passed through the stomach into the small bowel. These coatings work for some patients. On occasion, the coating never dissolves and the patient derives no benefit whatsoever from the drug; it passes unaltered into the toilet. On other occasions, the coating doesn't last long enough and nausea is encountered anyway.

Drugs are chemicals. Interactions between two drugs (two chemicals) are extremely common. Aspirin blocks absorption from the stomach of some of the newer anti-inflammatory agents discussed in the next section. Aspirin blocks the effects of probenecid on the excretion of uric acid. The world is complicated! By and large, the fewer medicines you take at one time, the more predictable your response to treatment will be. Most reactions having to do with absorption or interactions with other drugs are not perfectly predictable. You may have them or you may not. The treatment for your arthritis will ultimately be unique to you. You may need to discover by trial and error some of the reactions of your own body.

To figure things out for yourself, you must know about dosage equivalents, generic names, and product differences. Aspirin is huckstered more than any other drug. It is found in the drugstore in several hundred different formulations. It is "the drug doctors recommend most." Manufacturers compete to find tiny areas of difference between products in order to exploit these differences in advertising campaigns. There are "arthritis extra-strength" aspirins, buffered aspirins, and coated aspirins. There is aspirin with extra ingredients, such as caffeine or phenacetin. There is aspirin in cold formulations with antihistamines or other compounds. There is aspirin advertised for its purity.

A standard aspirin tablet is five grains, USP (*United States Pharmacopoeia*—the legal standard for drug strength and purity). This is 325 mg and the amount of drug is accurate to government standards. You always pay more for nonstandard aspirin formulations. For arthritis, do not buy aspirin that is compounded with any drugs other than possibly an antacid (Bufferin, Ascriptin). You do not want the caffeine, the phenacetin, or the antihistamine ingredients. Do not use a coated aspirin (Ecotrin, Enseals) unless you have stomach problems with a regular aspirin. They are more expensive and you may not get as good absorption from your stomach. Quality control is better on higher-priced aspirin (for example, Bayer), but few doctors believe that there is any additional therapeutic benefit. All of the USP aspirin are pure enough. So much for the science. If your body can tell a difference, stay with a product that seems to work for you. Otherwise, buy the cheapest USP aspirin that you can find. If it smells like vinegar when you open the bottle, it is too old. Throw it out.

The advice that follows is general advice. If your doctor's advice differs listen to your doctor. He or she is most familiar with your specific needs. The doses and precautions listed are those known at the time of this writing and are subject to changes your doctor may know about. But, if you receive advice that doesn't make sense according to the principles outlined here, don't hesitate to ask questions or get another opinion.

Aspirin (Acetosalicylic Acid)

Purpose: Mild pain reliever, major anti-inflammatory drug.

Indications: Pain relief for cartilage degeneration, local conditions. Anti-inflammatory agent for synovitis, attachment arthritis.

Dosage: For pain, two tablets (10 grains) every four hours as needed. For anti-inflammatory action, three to four tablets, four to six times daily with medical supervision if these doses are continued for longer than one week. The time to maximum effect is thirty minutes to one hour for pain and one to six weeks for the anti-inflammatory action.

Side effects: Common effects include nausea, vomiting, ringing in the ears, and decreased hearing. Each of these is reversible within a few hours if the drug dosage is decreased. Allergic reactions are rare but include development of nasal polyps and wheezing. Prolonged nausea or vomiting that persists after the drug is stopped for a few days suggests the possibility of a stomach ulcer caused by the irritation of the aspirin. With an overdose of aspirin, there is very rapid and heavy breathing, and there can even be unconsciousness and coma.

Aspirin has some predictable effects that occur in just about everyone but are quite well tolerated. Blood loss through the bowel occurs in almost all patients who take aspirin, because the platelet function is altered, the stomach is irritated, and aspirin acts as a minor blood-thinning agent. Up to 10 percent of patients taking high-dose aspirin will have some abnormalities in the function of the liver; although these are seldom noticed by the patient, they can be identified by blood tests. Since serious liver damage doesn't occur, routine blood tests to check for this complication are not required.

Special hints: If you note ringing in the ears or a decrease in your hearing, then decrease the dose of aspirin. You are just a little bit too high for the best result. If you notice nausea, an upset stomach, or vomiting, there are a variety of things you can do. First, try spreading out the dose with more frequent use of smaller numbers of pills. Perhaps instead of taking four tablets four times a day, you might take three tablets five or six times a day. Second, try taking the aspirin after meals or after an antacid, which will coat the stomach and provide some protection. Third, you can change brands and see if the nausea is related to the particular brand of aspirin you were using. Fourth, you can try coated aspirin. These are absorbed variably but are often effective at protecting the stomach and decreasing nausea. Ecotrin is the best absorbed and Enseals is next best. Probably other coated preparations should be avoided, since some of them are absorbed by very few people. You can drink 8 ounces of water after each dose to dilute the aspirin in the stomach. Finally, although it's a nuisance, you can get good relief from the nausea by taking a suspension of aspirin rather than the tablet. To do this, put the aspirin in a half glass of water and swirl it until the aspirin particles are suspended in the water. Fill another glass half full of water, drink the suspended aspirin and wash it down with the other glass of water. This is an effective and inexpensive way to avoid nausea once you get used to the taste.

Keep track of your aspirin intake and always tell your doctor how much you're taking. Aspirin is so familiar that sometimes we forget that we're taking a drug. Be as careful with aspirin as you would be with any prescription drug. In particular, you may want to ask your doctor about interactions with the newer anti-inflammatory agents, with probenecid, or with blood-thinning agents, if you are taking those drugs. Pay special attention to your stomach. So many drugs cause irritation to the stomach lining that you run the risk of adding insult to injury. Two drugs that irritate the stomach lining may be more than twice as dangerous; again, the fewer medications at one time the better.

Other Anti-inflammatory Agents that Are Not Steroids (NSAIA)

Aspirin is a *nonsteroidal anti-inflammatory agent*—that is, it is not a corticosteroid like prednisone, and it is an anti-inflammatory agent because it fights inflammation. Some of the disadvantages of aspirin have been noted above. In anti-inflammatory doses, side effects such as nausea, vomiting, and ringing in the ears are common. Some patients can't tolerate these side effects. Others, either ill-advised or not persistent, don't really try. Aspirin requires many tablets and regular attention to the medication schedule. So, a class of "aspirin substitutes," given the cumbersome name of nonsteroidal anti-inflammatory agents, has developed. In common medical usage, aspirin is not included in this group. To further simplify, we use the term *anti-inflammatory drugs* in this book. In the over-the-counter market, "aspirin substitute" usually refers to acetaminophen (Tylenol), which is discussed below as a pain reliever.

There is a huge market for drugs of this type. Nearly every drug company has tried to invent one and has promoted heavily whatever has been developed. Some of these drugs have been promoted in the financial pages of the newspaper or announced in press releases to the public before the scientific evidence was complete. Clearly, you have to be careful about what you read. But there is some substance to the claims. Many of these drugs are more consistently effective for attachment arthritis or for crystal arthritis than is aspirin. They may be better for those truly unable to tolerate aspirin. Unfortunately, they are more expensive, newer, and their long-term side effects are less well known. While present evidence suggests that they are slightly safer than aspirin because of fewer stomach problems, they probably should not be considered less hazardous yet. Aspirin has been used for centuries, whereas experience with these new drugs is sufficiently limited that some side effects may not yet have been discovered. They are useful drugs and rheumatologists are glad to be able to use them.

In perspective, the development of these drugs represents a substantial advance. In part, this is because of the difficult problems posed by the corticosteroids (discussed in the next section). The use of the term *nonsteroidal* to distinguish these compounds underscores the importance of this feature.

In anti-inflammatory potency, full doses of these drugs are roughly equivalent to full-dose aspirin or to about 10 to 15 mg per day of prednisone, a corticosteroid. Gastrointestinal side effects, such as heartburn and nausea, are usually less frequent than with aspirin—hence, an advantage for those with intolerant stomachs. Available evidence indicates that different drugs can be best for different individuals. These drugs come from several different chemical families and are not interchangeable. Patients may have to try several to find the most suitable one. The major medications in this category are discussed below. Throughout the chapter, the generic name of a drug is listed first, with its most common brand name in parentheses following.

Purpose: To reduce inflammation.

Indications: For reduction of inflammation in crystal arthritis, synovitis, attachment arthritis, local conditions, and more occasionally in cartilage degeneration.

Dosage: Three or four 100 mg capsules spread throughout the day. Short courses of treatment given for crystal arthritis or local conditions may be six capsules the first day, then five, four, three, two, and one on successive days for a six-day course.

Side effects: Unfortunately, these drugs can be hazardous. They were the first anti-inflammatory agents to be developed and our experience with them comprises some twenty years. We now know that on rare occasions they can cause serious problems with the blood, essentially killing all of the white cells or red cells. These conditions, termed *aplastic anemia* or *agranulocytosis,* can be fatal. They are very rare, occurring in perhaps one patient in every 10,000. When encountered, they are sometimes reversible after the drug is stopped, and they don't seem to occur if the drug is used only for a short period. Because if this toxicity, most doctors use the other drugs described below in preference to phenylbutazone (Butazolidine). This may be unfortunate, since phenylbutazone is a very effective medication in many instances. In crystal arthritis, a short course of this drug is often the most effective treatment available.

Irritation of the stomach lining also occurs, with nausea, heartburn, indigestion, and occasionally vomiting. Some patients retain fluid with phenylbutazone and a low salt diet is recommended. Allergic reactions, including rash, are rare.

Special hints: For nausea, spread the dose out a little through the day and take the capsules on a full stomach, perhaps one-half hour after meals. If you don't have a meal at that time, take an antacid half an hour before the medication. Occasional patients have better luck with oxyphenbutazone (Tandearil) if stomach upset with phenylbutazone is a major problem. Watch your weight; if it goes up, you are probably retaining fluid. If so, reduce the salt in your diet and be alert for any signs of shortness of breath. If shortness of breath occurs, call the doctor without delay.

While you are taking this drug, blood counts are recommended by most doctors, even though these tests don't protect you against the bad reaction. Possibly, however, they may enable an adverse reaction to be discovered more quickly. Blood counts every two weeks for the first three months and once a month thereafter are recommended by many doctors. For a short six-day course, no blood tests are required by most doctors. You should be able to tell if this is going to be a good drug for you within a week. If you haven't noticed major benefit, you may want to discuss a change in medication with your doctor.

Indomethacin (Indocin)

Purpose: To reduce inflammation, to slightly reduce pain.

Indications: To reduce inflammation in local conditions, attachment arthritis, crystal arthritis, synovitis, and sometimes cartilage degeneration.

Dosage: One 25 mg capsule three or four times daily. For men or large women, doses totaling as high as 150 to 200 mg (six to eight capsules) may be required and tolerated each day.

Side effects: Headache, slight dizziness, and a "spaced out" feeling are reported by many patients, particularly in the first few weeks of treatment. These tend to subside with continued treatment.

Irritation of the stomach lining, including nausea, indigestion, and heartburn, occurs with a number of patients. Allergic reaction including skin rash or asthma are very rare.

Special hints: This is one of the best drugs available for crystal arthritis and for attachment arthritis. In systemic lupus, it is often effective for some of the systemic problems, including inflammation of the lining of the lungs or heart. It is not consistently useful for synovitis and many doctors find it to be rather weak for treatment of rheumatoid arthritis in early stages, although it sometimes proves effective in later stages. In a long-term illness, maximum effect may take six weeks or so, but you should be able to tell within a week if the drug is going to be a major help.

There are some problems with absorption of indomethacin from the intestine. If you take it after meals, you have less stomach irritation, but some people don't absorb the drug very well. So, for maximum effect, you need to take it on an empty stomach and, for maximum comfort, to take it on a full stomach. Trial and error may be necessary to establish the best regimen for you. Aspirin poses another problem. When some individuals take aspirin with indomethacin, the indomethacin is not absorbed from the intestine. Usually you will not want to take these two drugs together, since you will get more irritation of the stomach lining but no more therapeutic effect than if you just took the aspirin. If this drug makes you feel mentally or emotionally fuzzy for more than the first few weeks, we think that is a good reason to discuss a change in medication with your doctor.

Ibuprofen (Motrin)

Purpose: To reduce inflammation, to slightly reduce pain.

Indications: For anti-inflammatory action in attachment arthritis, synovitis, local conditions, and occasionally degenerative cartilage changes.

Dosage: One or two 400 mg tablets three times daily. Maximum recommended dosage is 2400 mg, or eight tablets.

Side effects: Gastrointestinal side effects, with irritation of the stomach lining, are the most common, and include nausea, indigestion, and heartburn. Allergic reactions are rare and the drug is generally well tolerated. A very few patients, usually with lupus, have been observed who have had *aseptic meningitis* apparently related to this drug. Here, the patient experiences headache, fever, and stiff neck, and examination of the spinal fluid shows an increase in the protein and cells. The syndrome resolves when the drug is stopped, but can come back again if the drug is reintroduced. Occasionally, patients retain fluid with this medicine.

Special hints: Ibuprofen is not consistently useful for the treatment of synovitis. It turns out to be surprisingly useful in the treatment of attachment arthritis. Overall, many doctors are beginning to feel that it is one of the weaker therapeutic agents in this group. If you are not getting enough relief from it, you may wish to discuss a change in medication with your doctor. Avoidance of aspirin and other medications while taking Ibuprofen is advisable but not essential. It is absorbed reasonably well even on a full stomach, so if you have problems with irritation of the stomach take the drug after an antacid or after a meal. Maximum effect is achieved after about six weeks of treatment, but you should be able to see a major effect in the first week if it is going to be a really good drug for you.

Fenoprofen (Nalfon)

Purpose: To reduce inflammation, to slightly reduce pain.

Indications: For anti-inflammatory activity in synovitis, attachment arthritis, crystal arthritis, local conditions, and sometimes cartilage degeneration.

Dosage: One or two 300 mg capsules three or four times a day. Maximum recommended dosage is ten tablets daily.

Side effects: Irritation of the stomach lining is most frequent and includes nausea, indigestion, and heartburn. Allergic reactions including skin rash or asthma are very rare. Fluid retention is only very occasionally a problem.

Special hints: For stomach irritation, reduce the dose, by one or two tablets, spread it out throughout the day, or take the drug after meals or after antacid. Maximum effect may take six weeks or more, but you should see major benefit in the first week if the drug is going to be a great help to you. Aspirin should be avoided in general, although the evidence for its effect on the absorption of Fenoprofen is controversial. Fenoprofen is quite useful in synovitis and is preferred by many patients to aspirin on the basis of better effect on the disease as well as less bothersome side effects. It is reasonably good in attachment arthritis and has been useful in degenerative problems, particularly those involving the hip.

Naproxen (Naprosyn)

Purpose: To reduce inflammation, to slightly reduce pain.

Indications: For anti-inflammatory action in synovitis, attachment arthritis, crystal arthritis, local conditions, and sometimes cartilage degeneration.

Dosage: One 250 mg tablet twice a day or three times a day. Maximum recommended dosage is 750 mg (three tablets) a day.

Side effects: Gastrointestinal side effects, with irritation of the stomach lining, are the most common and include nausea, indigestion, and heartburn. Skin rash and other allergic problems are very rare. Fluid retention has been reported in a few individuals.

Special hints: Naproxen has an advantage over some other drugs of this class in having a longer "half-life." Thus, you don't have to take as many tablets as with the other medicines in this group. Each tablet lasts from eight to twelve hours. In general, aspirin should be avoided, since it interferes with Naproxen in some individuals. If you notice fluid retention, reduce your salt intake and discuss a change in medication with your doctor. Naproxen (Naprosyn) is liked by many patients because of the small number of tablets required. It is quite effective in synovitis such as rheumatoid arthritis and is preferred by some patients over aspirin and other drugs of this group. It is consistently effective in attachment arthritis and is preferred by many patients with this problem. Degenerative arthritis of the hip also responds to the drug, and a few physicians use it for crystal-arthritis control. If you have stomach irritation, try taking the tablets on a full stomach or after antacids. Although absorption may be slightly decreased, you may be more comfortable overall.

Tolmetin (Tolectin)

Purpose: To reduce inflammation, to reduce pain slightly.

Indications: For anti-inflammatory activity in synovitis, attachment arthritis, local conditions, crystal arthritis, and occasionally degenerative arthritis.

Dosage: Two 200 mg tablets three or four times daily. Maximum recommended dosage is 2000 mg, or ten tablets.

Side effects: The most frequent side effects are gastrointestinal, as with other drugs of this group. Irritation of the stomach lining can cause nausea, heartburn, and indigestion. Occasionally patients note fluid retention. Allergic reactions such as rash or asthma are very rare.

Special hints: For irritation of the stomach, decrease the dose or spread out the tablets throughout the day. Absorption will be slightly decreased if you take the drug after meals or after antacids, but greater comfort may result. Aspirin and other drugs of this class may potentially interfere with absorption and the best rule is to take just one drug at a time. Tolmetin is useful in synovitis, such as rheumatoid arthritis, and in attachment arthritis. It has found use in degenerative arthritis of the hip and for treatment of local conditions. As with other drugs of this group, certain patients will prefer Tolmetin to all other drugs of the group.

Sulindac (Clinoril)

Purpose: To reduce inflammation, to reduce pain slightly.

Indications: For anti-inflammatory action in attachment arthritis, synovitis, gout, local conditions, and occasionally, degenerative cartilage changes.

Dosage: One 150 mg tablet twice a day. This drug also comes in a 200 mg tablet and dosage may be increased to 200 mg twice a day if needed. Maximum recommended dose is 400 mg a day.

Side effects: Gastro-intestinal side effects, with irritation of the stomach lining, are the most common, and include nausea, indigestion, and heartburn. Stomach pain has been reported in ten percent of subjects, and nausea, diarrhea, constipation, headache, and rash in from three to nine percent. Ringing in the ears, fluid retention, itching, and nervousness have been reported. A few patients have had bleeding from the stomach. Allergic reactions are rare. The use of aspirin in combination with this drug is not recommended by the manufacturer, since aspirin apparently decreases absorption from the intestine.

Special hints: Sulindac has no particular advantages or disadvantages compared with the anti-inflammatory agents described above. It was introduced in October of 1978 with great fanfare. Announcement of its availability was made through press releases, creating public expectation that a major advance in treatment of arthritis had occurred. No mention was made that other agents were already available which did everything that Clinoril does. Studies over the past several years have indicated that no major advance is represented by this drug. It may be useful in some patients. But, since Nalfon, Motrin, Naprosyn, Tolectin, and Indocin have been around longer, they have a greater proven safety record and should be used first. Indocin is made by the same manufacturer and is much cheaper; the Indocin patent is about to expire, and indomethacin will become cheaper yet. At this writing, Clinoril is the most expensive of the anti-inflammatory agents.

I am disturbed by the raising of false hopes with new drug introductions. This had occurred with the introduction of Motrin, Naprosyn, and others, but the Clinoril example is the most recent and most pronounced. Each physician seeing patients with arthritis was bombarded by patient requests to try the new drug. Disappointment followed for many, and sound treatment practices may have been interrupted.

For stomach upset, take the pills after meals; skip a dose or two if necessary. Antacids may be used for gastrointestinal problems and may sometimes help. Check with your doctor if the distress continues. Maximum therapeutic effect is achieved after about six weeks of treatment, but you should be able to see a major effect in the first week if Clinoril is going to be a really good drug for you.

Corticosteroids

In about 1950, a widely heralded miracle occurred—the introduction of cortisone for the treatment of arthritis. The Nobel prize was awarded to the doctors who developed this drug. Patients with rheumatoid arthritis and other forms of synovitis suddenly noted that the swelling and pain in their joints decreased and that the overall toxicity of the disease disappeared. They felt fine.

The initial enthusiasm for cortisone in arthritis was tremendous. But, over the years, a number of major cautions began to be voiced. Slowly, the cumulative side effects of the cortisonelike drugs began to be recognized. For many patients, the side effects were clearly greater than any benefits obtained. Cortisone became the model of a drug that provides early benefits but late penalties. Now, with a quarter of a century of experience behind us, our perspective is more complete. Such drugs represent a major treatment for arthritis, but their use is appropriate in only a relatively small number of patients and then only with full attention to potential complications.

Steroids are natural hormones manufactured by the adrenal glands. When used medically, they are given in doses somewhat higher than the amounts the body generally makes. In these doses they suppress the function of your own adrenal glands and lead to a kind of drug dependency as the gland slowly shrinks. After many months of steroid use, the drug must be withdrawn slowly to allow your own adrenal glands to return to full function, otherwise an "adrenal crisis" can occur in which you don't have enough hormone. Steroids must be taken exactly as directed and a physician's close supervision is always required.

Let's discuss the side effects. They can be divided into categories depending on the length of time you have been taking the steroid and the dose prescribed. Side effects result from a combination of how high the dose is and how long you have been taking it. If you have been taking steroids for less than one week, side effects are quite rare even if the dose has been high.

If you have been taking high doses for one week to one month, you are at risk for development of ulcers, mental changes including psychosis or depression, infection with bacterial germs, or acne over the skin. The side effects of steroids are most apparent between one month and one year of medium-to-high-dose steroid. The patient becomes fat in the central parts of the body, with a buffalo hump on the lower neck and wasting of the muscles in the arms and legs. Hair growth increases over the face, skin bruises appear, and stretch marks develop over the abdomen. After years of steroid treatment (even with low doses) there is a loss of calcium, resulting in fragile bones. Even slight injuries can cause fractures. Cataracts develop slowly and the skin becomes thin and translucent. Some physicians believe that hardening of the arteries occurs more rapidly and that there may be complications of inflammation of the arteries.

Many of these side effects will occur in everyone who takes sufficient doses of cortisone or its drug relatives for a sufficient period of time, but there are some tricks that help. The art of managing arthritis with corticosteroids involves knowing how to minimize these side effects. The physician will work with you to keep the dose as low as possible at all times. If possible, you may be instructed to take the drug only once daily rather than several times daily, since there are fewer side effects when it is taken this way. If you are able to tolerate the drug only every other day, this is even better for the side effects are then quite minimal. Unfortunately, some patients find that the dosage schedules that cause the fewest side effects also give them the least relief.

I very seldom use corticosteroids for arthritis alone, although I use them relatively frequently in the connective-tissue diseases. Always they are used with great respect and caution. Some experienced doctors use low-dose corticosteroid treatment in rheumatoid arthritis more than I do, demonstrating that the proper indications for use of these drugs still is somewhat controversial. High-dose cortisone treatment for uncomplicated rheumatoid arthritis has long been considered bad practice in the United States; it remains the essence of some quack treatments of arthritis, such as those available in Mexican border towns or Canada (Liefcort). Corticosteroids are not useful in attachment arthritis or generalized conditions. They are harmful in infectious arthritis and should not be given by mouth in local conditions or cartilage degeneration.

There are three ways to give corticosteroids. They can be taken by mouth, they can be given by injection into the painful area, or an injection of adrenal cortical stimulating hormone (ACTH) can be given to cause the patient's own adrenal gland to increase production of hormones. Prednisone (or prednisolone) is the steroid usually given by mouth and is the reference steroid discussed here. There are perhaps twenty different steroid drugs now available. Cortisone itself retains too much fluid and the second drug developed, hydrocortisone, has the same deficit. The fluorinated steroids, such as triamcinolone, cause greater problems with muscle wasting than does prednisone. The steroids sold by brand name are about twenty times as expensive as prednisone and do not have any major advantages. Hence, there is little reason to use any of these other compounds for administration of steroids by mouth.

Prednisone

Purpose: To reduce inflammation, to suppress immunological responses.

Indications: For suppression of muscle inflammation and serious systemic manifestations of connective-tissue diseases, such as kidney involvement. Occasionally, for use in suppressing the inflammation of synovitis.

Dosage: The normal body makes the equivalent of about 5 to 7.5 mg of prednisone each day. "Low-dose" prednisone treatment is from 5 to 10 mg. "Moderate-dose" ranges from 15 to 30 mg per day and "high-dose" from 40 to 60 mg per day, or even higher. The drug is often most effective when given in several doses throughout the day, but side effects are least when the same total daily dose is given as infrequently as possible.

Side effects: Prednisone causes all of the side effects of the corticosteroids listed above. Allergy is extremely rare. Side effects are related to dose and to duration of treatment. The side effects are major and include fatal complications. Psychological dependency often occurs and complicates efforts to get off of the drug once you have begun.

Special hints: Discuss the need for prednisone very carefully with your doctor before beginning. The decision to start steroid treatment for a chronic disease is a major one and you want to be sure that the drug is essential. You may want a second opinion if the explanation does not completely satisfy you. When taking prednisone, follow your doctor's instructions very closely. With some drugs it doesn't make much difference if you start and stop them on your own, but prednisone must be taken extremely regularly and exactly as prescribed. You will want to help your doctor decrease your dose of prednisone whenever possible, even if this does cause some increase in your symptoms.

A funny thing happens when you reduce the dose of prednisone: a syndrome called *steroid fibrositis* can cause increased stiffness and pain for a week or ten days after each dose reduction. Sometimes this is interpreted as return of the arthritis and the opportunity to reduce the dose of prednisone is lost. If you are going to take prednisone for a long time, ask your doctor about taking some vitamin D along with it. There is some evidence, still controversial, that the loss of bone, the most critical long-term side effect, can be reduced if you take vitamin D.

If you are having some side effects, ask your doctor about once daily or every-other-day use of the prednisone. Watch your salt intake and keep it low, since there is a slight tendency to retain fluid with prednisone. Watch your diet as well, since you will be fighting an increase in appetite and a tendency to put on unseemly fat. If you stay active and limit the calories you take in, you can minimize many of the ugly side effects of the steroid medication and can improve the strength of the bones and the muscles. If you are taking a corticosteroid other than prednisone by mouth, ask your physician if it is all right to switch to the equivalent dose of prednisone.

Steroid Injections (Triamcinalone Hexacetonide; Depo-Medrol; Many Others)

Purpose: To reduce inflammation in a local area by injection into that area.

Indications: Noninfectious inflammation and pain in a particular region of the body. Or a widespread arthritis with one or two areas causing most of the problem.

Dosage: This varies depending on the preparation and purpose desired. Frequency of injection is more important. Usually injections should not be repeated more frequently than each six weeks and only a limited number of injections should be given to a single area.

Side effects: Steroid injections resemble a very short course of prednisone by mouth and therefore have few side effects. They result in a high concentration of the steroid in the area that is inflamed and can have quite a pronounced effect in reducing this inflammation. If a single area is injected many times, the injection appears to cause damage in that area. This has resulted in serious problems in frequently injected areas, such as the elbows of baseball pitchers. Some studies suggest that as few as ten injections can cause increased bone destruction; hence, most doctors stop injecting before this time.

Special hints: If one area of your body is giving you a lot of trouble, an injection frequently makes sense. The response to the first injection will tell you quite accurately how much sense it makes. If you get excellent relief that lasts for many months, reinjection is indicated if the problem returns. The steroid injections contain a "long-acting" steroid, but it is only in the body for a few days. Effects may last much longer than this, since the injection may break a cycle of inflammation and injury. If you get relief but it lasts only for a few days, then injection is not going to be a very useful treatment for you. If you get no relief at all or an increase in pain, this is an obvious sign that other kinds of treatment should be sought. If a joint which bears weight has been injected, be gentle with the weight-bearing for a few days. If you can find a "trigger point" on your body where pressure reproduces your major pain, then injection of the trigger point is frequently beneficial. Occasionally, patients with degenerative arthritis get benefit from injections, but usually injections are not helpful unless there is inflammation in the area.

ACTH (Adrenocortical Stimulating Hormone)

Purpose: To reduce inflammation.

Indications: Probably none.

Dosage: Variable.

Side effects: Repeated injections cause all the side effects noted in the general discussion above. Occasional injections cause local pain but few other problems.

Special hints: This method of administering corticosteroids is now practiced by very few physicians. It is not that it is bad as much as that it has been superseded by less expensive and less cumbersome methods of treatment. With ACTH injections, you get an increased dose of corticosteroids manufactured by your own body, principally cortisone and hydrocortisone. These higher doses cause more salt retention than you get with oral prednisone. Moreover, you and your doctor don't know exactly what dose you are getting. It depends on the state of your own adrenal glands at the time of the injection. Thus, the same injection for different patients may result in widely varying doses of cortisone. Further, it is painful and expensive. Some doctors use ACTH injections to "wake up" a patient's own adrenal gland after it has been suppressed by a long period of prednisone administration. Unfortunately, there is little evidence that this speeds up the process of rejuvenation of one's own adrenal gland, which may take months anyway. So, I don't see much rationale for this kind of treatment and I never use it. A few doctors still do and, if you can afford it, no great harm has been done.

Antimalarial Drugs

For mysterious reasons, the chloroquine family of drugs works in reducing the inflammation of synovitis and can also decrease the skin problems of lupus. These drugs were developed for control of malaria and have been widely used around the world for this purpose. Chloroquine and hydroxychloroquine (Plaquenil) are the most frequently used drugs of this class. They accumulate slowly in the body, particularly in the cells of the body that contain pigment. Their effectiveness in rheumatoid arthritis and in lupus has been well proven. After stopping the drug, the drug remains in the body for many months before slowly being eliminated.

These drugs are superbly tolerated and cause few noticeable side effects. Unfortunately, the remote possibility of blindness must be included in the list of possible side effects. Eye changes include reversible minor changes in the front of the eyes and more serious, sometimes irreversible changes in the pigmented area in the back of the eye. This side effect, called *macular degeneration,* may be aggravated by bright sunlight which is focused on the pigment-containing cells. Side effects in the stomach or bowel are rare and muscle weakness is sometimes reported but is very rare. The safety of these drugs is exemplified by the fact that they have been used for malaria prevention around the world in many millions of individuals. While the doses used for treatment of arthritis are slightly higher than those which prevent malaria, the safety record is still very good.

The effects of these drugs are consistent although not often dramatic, and they work well together with aspirin or other anti-inflammatory agents. There are no known drug interactions involving these drugs. In the past, atabrine and other antimalarial drugs were used as well. Atabrine is now used rarely, because it turns the skin yellow as it accumulates in the skin. Hydroxychloroquine is generally believed to have fewer eye side effects than chloroquine and is the most commonly recommended drug at the present time.

Hydroxychloroquine (Plaquenil); Chloroquine

Purpose: To reduce inflammation in synovitis.

Indications: Synovitis or the skin lesions of lupus.

Dosage: Hydroxychloroquine—one or two 200 mg tablets daily (200–400 mg). Chloroquine—one or two 250 mg tablets once daily (250–500 mg).

Side effects: Rare. Because of the possibility of eye damage, an ophthalmologist should check the eyes after nine months of treatment and at three to six-month intervals thereafter. Eye damage is rare and appears to be reversible in most instances when detected sufficiently early. It occurs slowly and has not yet been reported before nine months of treatment. Some physicians request an eye examination before even prescribing one of these drugs; others believe that the safety record of Plaquenil is so good that no formal eye examinations are required.

Special hints: Don't expect to feel any change immediately after taking these drugs. It takes six to twelve weeks for the effect to become apparent and it will come on so gradually that many people aren't sure that it is really a drug effect or if they are just getting better by themselves. Similarly, when you stop the drug, the beneficial effect may linger for a number of weeks before gradually going away. These drugs are very slowly accumulated and very slowly excreted.

The biggest reason why these drugs aren't used more widely is the trouble and expense of the eye examinations. When these tests are included in the cost, antimalarial drugs become expensive treatments. However, you do get a free trial. You can begin the drug without any eye examination to determine first whether it will be good for you or not. If after several months there is no sign of improvement, you can then discontinue the drug well before any eye problem. On the other hand, if you are getting benefit, then it will be worth having the eye tests. I use these drugs quite a bit and have yet to see my first case of any eye toxicity. Often in medicine it happens that very unlikely events cause the greatest concern and so it is with the eye problems of hydroxychloroquine and chloroquine.

Gold Salts and Penicillamine

These are major-league drugs, although no one knows why they are so effective in so many patients. They provide dramatic benefits to over two-thirds of patients with severe synovitis. Each has major side effects that require stopping treatment in at least one-quarter of patients and, infrequently, may even be fatal. Gold salts and penicillamine are two very different kinds of drugs, but there are striking similarities in the type and magnitude of good effects and in the type of side effects. Neither appears to be of use in any category other than synovitis, but the scientific proof of their effectiveness in synovitis is impressive.

These agents can result in remission. In perhaps one-quarter of patients, the disease will actually be so well controlled that neither doctor nor patient can find any evidence of it. Usually these drugs have to be continued in order to maintain the remission, but the effects can be more dramatic than with any other agent to reduce inflammation, except possibly some of the immunosuppressant drugs discussed below. Patients using these drugs must accept certain significant hazards, but there is a good chance of very major benefit. In rheumatoid arthritis, these drugs have been proven to slow down the process of joint destruction.

If you are not able to tolerate one of these drugs, you may be able to tolerate the other. If you don't get a good response from one, you may from the other. After failure with one drug, the chances decrease a little, but success with the second drug is still common.

Which should be tried first? No one knows. In England, penicillamine is usually used first. In the United States, it is gold. Gold must be given by injection and requires a doctor visit every week for a while. With costs of blood tests, the total dollar cost of the initial course may be $800.

Penicillamine can be taken by mouth and, while the drug itself is expensive, the total cost may be less because of slightly fewer blood tests. At this writing, penicillamine has just become officially approved in the United States for arthritis treatment. In terms of effectiveness and risk, you can consider these two drugs about the same.

Gold Salts (Myochrysine, Solganal)

Purpose: To reduce inflammation.

Indications: Synovitis that is not responsive to less hazardous medications or is severe and rapidly progressive.

Dosage: 50 mg per week by intramuscular injection for twenty weeks, then one to two injections per month thereafter. Many doctors use smaller doses for the first two injections to test for allergic reactions to the injections. Sometimes doctors give more or less than this standard dosage depending on your body size and response to treatment. "Maintenance" gold treatment refers to injections after the first twenty weeks (which result in 1,000 mg of total gold). The dosage and duration of maintenance therapy varies quite a bit; with good responses, the gold maintenance may be continued for many years, with injections given every two to six weeks.

Side effects: The gold salts accumulate very slowly in the tissues of the joints and in other parts of the body. Hence, side effects usually occur only after a considerable amount of gold has been received, although allergic reactions can occur even with the initial injection. The major side effects have to do with the skin, the kidneys, and the blood cells. The skin can develop a rash, usually occurring after ten or more injections, with big red spots or blotches, often itchy. If the rash remains a minor problem, the drug may be cautiously continued, but occasionally a very serious rash occurs following gold injections.

The kidney can be damaged so that protein leaks out of the body through the urine. This is called *nephrosis* or the *nephrotic syndrome* if it is severe. When it is recognized and the drug is stopped, the nephrosis usually goes away, but cases have been reported in which it did not reverse. The blood-cell problems are the most dangerous. They can affect either the white blood cells or the platelets, those blood cells that control the clotting of the blood. In each case, the gold causes the bone marrow to stop making the particular blood cell. If the white cells are not made, the body becomes susceptible to serious infections that can be fatal. If the platelets are not made, the body is subject to serious bleeding episodes that can be fatal. Stopping the drug almost always reverses these problems, but reversal may take several weeks, during which the patient is at risk for a major medical problem.

Other potential side effects, such as ulcers in the mouth, a mild hepatitis, or nausea, usually are not as troublesome. Overall, about one-quarter of patients have to stop their course of treatment because of the side effects. One or two percent of patients experience a significant side effect; the other patients won't really notice very much of a problem, even though they may be on the verge of a serious side effect. About one in a thousand times, there may be a fatal side effect. With careful monitoring, the drug is reasonably safe and its benefits justify its use, since over 70 percent of patients treated with gold show moderate or marked improvement. However, you must maintain your respect for this treatment and keep up regular blood tests to detect early side effects. One final note: Most but not all side effects occur during the first induction period of twenty injections.

Special hints: You must learn to be patient with gold treatment. The gold accumulates slowly in the body and its good effects are almost never observed in the first ten weeks of treatment. Improvement begins slowly after that and major improvement is usually evident by the end of 1,000 mg, or twenty weeks. Similarly, if the drug is stopped, it requires many months before the effect is totally lost. In one famous study, the gold group was still doing better than the control group two years after the drug had been discontinued, although most of the effect of the drug had been lost by that time. After a side effect, many doctors will suggest that the drug be tried again. Often, this can be worthwhile if the approach is very cautious, since the drug is frequently tolerated the second time around. We do not try gold salts again if there has been a problem with the blood, but will use it again cautiously after mild skin reactions or mild amounts of protein loss through the urine.

To minimize the chance of serious side effects, most doctors recommend that a check be made of the urine for protein leakage, and of the white cells and the platelets. Further, before every injection, the patient should be questioned about skin rash. This is good practice. Unfortunately, the combination of twenty doctor visits, twenty injections, twenty urinalyses, twenty blood counts, and so forth, makes the cost of initiating gold treatment approximately $800 when pursued in this manner. There are some ways to decrease this cost while preserving safeguards. You can ask your doctor to prescribe some test materials, so that you can test your urine for protein at home. This is a very easy technique. You can ask if it is possible to have just a platelet smear and a white count rather than a complete blood count each time. You can inquire whether it is possible to have the nurse give an injection after checking the blood counts without actually having a doctor visit every week. A few patients have even successfully given their own shots at home with the help of their family, although this is not acceptable to many. By using such techniques, you can save half to three-quarters of the cost of a course of gold treatment.

Penicillamine (Cuprimine)

Purpose: To reduce inflammation.

Indications: Synovitis that is not responsive to less hazardous medications or is severe and rapidly progressive.

Dosage: Usually 250 mg (one tablet) per day for a month, then two tablets (500 mg) a day for a month, then three tablets (750 mg) for a month, and finally in some patients to four tablets (1,000 mg) per day. After a successful remission, this dosage, or a lower one, can be continued indefinitely.

Side effects: These closely follow those noted above for gold injections. The major side effects are skin rash, protein leakage through the urine, or a decrease in production of the blood cells. Additionally, patients may have nausea, and many patients notice a metallic taste in the mouth or a decreased sense of taste. Penicillamine weakens the connective tissue so that the healing of a cut is delayed, and a scar may not have the same strength it would have without the penicillamine. So, stitches following a cut should be left in for a longer period of time, and wound healing should be expected to be delayed. Surgery under these circumstances may be more difficult.

Special hints: Penicillamine takes a number of months to reach its therapeutic effect and the effect persists for a long time after you stop taking the drug. Responses usually take between three to six months, but can be as late as nine months after the drug is begun. Because of the risk of side effects, doctors have in general adopted the "go low, go slow" approach suggested in the dosage schedule above. When full doses were begun earlier, the frequency of side effects was higher. Even now, only about three-quarters of patients will complete the treatment and the remainder will have some side effects, approximately the same as those listed for gold salts. The drug may be tried again after a side effect if the side effect has been mild. We do not use the drug again if there has been a problem with the blood counts, but may cautiously try it if there has been a minor problem with protein in the urine or a minor skin rash or minor nausea.

Monitoring for side effects has to be carefully performed. Usually a blood count or smear, a urinalysis for protein, and questioning of the patient for side effects are required every two weeks or even more frequently. It should be noted that with both penicillamine and gold, careful monitoring improves your chances of not having a serious side effect, but does not eliminate them. These drugs contain hazards that no physician can entirely eliminate. Again, you can negotiate to have some of the drug monitoring done by a local laboratory and review the results yourself, check your own urine for protein, and so forth, if you desire. Most doctors who use these drugs a good deal have evolved some method of minimizing the cost of the monitoring. Again, after the first six months, side effects are relatively rare but still do occur. Some patients have an excellent response to the penicillamine even though they never get up to the full dosage of 1,000 mg per day.

DRUGS TO REDUCE PAIN

This section is included mainly to emphasize that pain-reducing drugs have little place in the treatment of arthritis. Consider their four major disadvantages. First, they don't do anything for the arthritis, they just cover it up. Second, they help defeat the pain mechanism that tells you when you are doing something that is injuring your body. If you suppress it, you may injure your body without being aware of it. Third, the body adjusts to pain medicines, so they aren't very effective over the long term. This phenomenon is called *tolerance* and develops to some extent with all of the drugs we commonly use. Fourth, pain medicines can have major side effects. The side effects range from stomach distress to constipation to mental changes. Most of these drugs are "downers," which you don't need if you have arthritis. You need to be able to cope with a somewhat more difficult living situation than the average person. These drugs decrease your ability to solve problems.

Many patients develop a tragic dependence on these agents. In arthritis, the addiction is somewhat different than what we usually imagine. Most patients with arthritis are not physically addicted to codeine or Percodan or Demerol. They are psychologically dependent on these drugs as a crutch and become inordinately concerned with an attempt to eliminate every last symptom. These agents conflict with the attempt to achieve independent living for the patient with arthritis.

By and large, use these drugs only for the short term and only when resting the sore part, so that you don't reinjure it while the pain is suppressed. Drugs mentioned first in this section are less harmful than those listed later. Drugs to reduce inflammation, discussed in the previous section, may reduce pain through direct pain action as well as through reduction of inflammation. This is preferable.

These same principles hold for a number of less common pain relievers not described here.

Acetaminophen (Tylenol, Other Brands)

Purpose: For temporary relief of minor pain.

Indications: Mild temporary pain, particularly cartilage degeneration.

Dosage: Two tablets (10 grains) every four hours as needed.

Side effects: Minimal. Unlike aspirin, acetaminophen usually does not upset the stomach, does not cause ringing in the ears, does not affect the clotting of the blood, does not interact with other medications, and is about as safe as can be. Of course, as with any drug, occasional problems arise, but this drug is frequently recommended in place of aspirin for children because of its greater safety.

Special hints: Acetaminophen is not anti-inflammatory; thus it is not an aspirin substitute in the treatment of arthritis. If the condition is not an inflammatory one, then it may be approximately as useful as aspirin with fewer side effects. It is only a mild pain reliever and therefore has fewer disadvantages than the following agents. It is relatively inexpensive.

Purpose: Mild pain relief.

Indications: For short-term use in decreasing mild pain.

Dosage: One-half grain (32 mg) or one grain (65 mg) every four hours as needed for pain.

Side effects: These drugs are widely promoted and widely used with a reasonably good safety record. In some cases, side effects may be due to the aspirin or other medication in combination with the Darvon. Most worrisome to us has been the mentally dull feeling that many patients report, sometimes described as being a grey, semiunhappy fog. Other patients don't seem to notice this effect. Side reactions include dizziness, headache, sedation, somnolence, excitement, skin rash, and gastrointestinal disturbances. These drugs are often involved in suicide attempts and sometimes actual suicides.

Special hints: Darvon is not anti-inflammatory and is thus not an aspirin substitute. The pain relief given is approximately equal to aspirin in most cases. The drug is more expensive than aspirin or acetaminophen. It does come in a pretty capsule, shaped rather like a bullet.

Codeine (Empirin #1, 2, 3, 4, ASA with Codeine #1, 2, 3, 4)

Purpose: Moderate pain relief.

Indications: For moderate pain relief over the short term.

Dosage: For some curious reason, the strengths of codeine are often coded in numbers. For example, Empirin with codeine #1 or just Empirin #1 contains one-eighth grain or 8 mg of codeine per tablet, #2 contains one-fourth grain or 16 mg, #3 contains one-half grain or 32 mg, and #4 contains one grain or 65 mg of codeine phosphate. A common dosage is a #3 tablet (32 mg codeine) every four hours as needed for pain.

Side effects: The side effects are proportional to the dosage. The more you take, the more side effects you are likely to have. Allergic reactions are quite rare.
  Codeine is a narcotic. Thus, it can lead to addiction, with tolerance and drug dependence. Frequently in arthritis patients it leads to constipation and sometimes a set of complications including fecal impaction and diverticuli. More worrisome to us is the way that patients on codeine seem to lose their will to cope. The patient taking codeine for many years sometimes seems sluggish and generally depressed. We don't really know if the codeine is responsible, but we do think that codeine often makes it more difficult for the patient with arthritis to cope with the very real problems that abound.

Oxycodone (Percodan, Percobarb, Percogesic)

Purpose: For pain relief. Not generally a drug for arthritis.

Indications: For short-term relief of severe pain, as with a broken bone or recent surgery.

Dosage: One tablet every six hours as needed.

Side effects: Percodan is a curious combination drug. The basic narcotic is oxycodone, to which is added aspirin and other minor pain relievers. Combination drugs have a number of theoretical disadvantages, but Percodan is a strong and effective reliever of pain. It does require a special prescription because it is a strong narcotic and the hazards of serious addiction are present. The manufacturers state that the habit-forming potentialities are somewhat less than morphine and somewhat greater than codeine. The drug is usually well tolerated.

Special hints: Percodan is a good drug for people with cancer, but we don't find much use for it in treatment of arthritis. It is not an anti-inflammatory agent and does not directly work on any of the disease processes. It is habit forming and it does break the pain reflex. It is a mental depressant and serious addiction can result.

Demerol

Purpose: For relief of severe pain. Not a drug for arthritis.

Indications: For temporary relief of severe pain, as with a bad fracture that has been immobilized.

Dosage: Various preparations come with 25 mg, 50 mg, or 100 mg of demerol. One tablet every four hours for pain is a typical dose. Dose is increased for more severe pain and decreased for milder pain.

Side effects: This is a major narcotic approximately equivalent to morphine in pain relief and in addiction potential. Tolerance develops and increasing doses may be required. Drug dependence and severe withdrawal symptoms may be seen if the drug is stopped. Psychological dependence also occurs. The underlying disease may be covered up and serious symptoms may be masked. Nausea, vomiting, constipation, and a variety of other side effects may occur.

Special hints: I have never used this drug for arthritis. The several times I have seen others use it for arthritis, the consequences have been disastrous. It is not a drug for treatment of arthritis. Stay away from it.

This discussion is about drugs for gout. Pseudogout and the other rare forms of crystal arthritis do just about as well with the anti-inflammatory drugs described earlier. There is no problem with uric acid with pseudogout. This section therefore focuses on three types of drug used almost exclusively in the treatment of gout.

Think about the four stages of gout. First, there is pre-gout, in which there is a metabolic disturbance (elevation of uric acid), but no disease. An attack of gouty arthritis may follow. Then there is an interval during which the patient is free of symptoms. Finally, there may be an accumulation of uric acid around the joints, so-called tophaceous gout.

To treat gout, you use different drugs for different stages. Most people with the first stage will not get the second. Most with the second will not get the last. The first stage does not require treatment. To stop the acute attack, we generally use colchicine or one of the drugs that reduce inflammation. The nonsteroidal anti-inflammatory agents are all effective at this second stage. During interval gout, we may use probenecid to reduce the uric acid. If we want to reduce uric acid in the urine as well, so as to prevent or decrease the chance of kidney stones, we use allopurinol. In tophaceous gout we use probenecid, allopurinol, or both.

Management of gout in all of its stages should be precise, since this is a disease subject to the laws of physics that govern crystal formation. Still, this condition is managed incorrectly as frequently as it is managed correctly. There are nine commonly made mistakes. Avoid these problems and you will do well.

- **Overtreatment of elevated uric acid.** An elevated uric acid should almost never be treated if it has not caused any problems. The same holds if diuretic drugs have caused the raised uric acid without consequent problems. There are side effects of treatment, and a lifetime of treatment may cost as much as $20,000 in accumulated medical costs. There are no proven medical benefits. Enough said.

- **Combination of aspirin and probenecid.** The aspirin prevents the probenecid from working. Tylenol may be used in place of aspirin for headaches and the like.

- **Using diuretics in patients with gout.** Diuretics *increase* the uric acid and may cause some acute attacks of gout. They should be avoided when possible.

- **Combination of allopurinol (Zyloprim) and azathioprine (Imuran).** There can be fatal side effects from the use of these two drugs together, since the allopurinol greatly increases the toxicity of the azathioprine. They should *never* be used in combination. The same is true of 6-mercaptopurine (6-MP) and allopurinol.

- **Use of allopurinol for acute gout attacks.** This is simply wrong. Allopurinol does not treat *acute* gouty arthritis and may in fact make it worse.

- **Use of probenecid for gout attacks.** Wrong again. This is not a treatment for gouty arthritis. Probenecid lowers the uric acid but does nothing for the *acute* attack.

- **Use of probenecid for patients with kidney stones.** Unfortunately, probenecid *increases* the chances of kidney stones, at least temporarily. It causes an increased elimination of uric acid through the kidneys and the uric acid may collect to form the stone.

- **Use of colchicine to lower uric acid.** Another wrong concept. Colchicine has no effect on the uric-acid level.

- **Reliance on drugs to the exclusion of other treatments.** Weight control, regular exercise, minimization of stress, decrease in certain dietary components, and other measures including high fluid intake are important for management of gout. Because we have strong drugs to manage this condition, we have tended to rely on those rather than on the nondrug treatments. But drugs are expensive and have the possibility of harm. There are additional health benefits from control of these other factors and they must not be neglected.

Colchicine

Purpose: For gout attacks and to prevent acute gouty arthritis.

Indication: Gout attack or, for preventive therapy, a history of an attack of gout.

Dosage: For prevention, one 0.6 mg tablet twice daily is the usual dose. For treatment of the acute attack, the medication may be given either by mouth or intravenously. By mouth the usual dosage is one 0.6 mg tablet every hour until relief is obtained, side effects such as diarrhea are noticed, or a total of eight to twelve tablets is reached. When given by vein, 2 mg is the usual dose, and many doctors do not like to exceed 3 mg in any 24-hour period.

Side effects: These can get pretty impressive. When you are taking a tablet of colchicine every hour for an acute attack, you usually begin to experience relief after about six to eight hours. At the same time, the diarrhea begins and the diarrhea and accompanying stomach cramps make some patients wish that they had their acute gouty arthritis back again and were rid of the diarrhea. So, the minute you note the slightest sign of diarrhea, stop there.

Colchicine, when taken for preventive purposes, has almost no side effects, because the dosage is lower.

Intravenous colchicine is usually well tolerated. There have been deaths reported from treatment with intravenous colchicine in hospitalized patients and this has happened with as little as 7 to 10 mg of the drug in ten hours. For this reason, many doctors keep an absolute limit of 3 mg of intravenous drug. As far as can be told, the drug is safe when used in this more moderate dosage. There is no diarrhea when the drug is taken by vein.

Special hints: The advantage of colchicine over the nonsteroidal agents for the treatment of acute gout is the diagnostic assistance it affords. Colchicine is good for gout attacks, but it is essentially worthless in other kinds of arthritis. So, if the doctor doesn't know what kind of arthritis you have, giving cochicine can help make that determination. If you respond, it's gout; if you don't it probably isn't.

As noted, the side effects of colchicine can be rather distressing. Certainly colchicine by mouth is much more uncomfortable for the patient than is Indocin, Naprosyn, Nalfon, Motrin, phenylbutazone, ACTH, or corticosteroids. Each of these other drugs can be useful in treating the acute attack and, after the first attack, you should usually be on one of them instead of colchicine. My own preference is for phenylbutazone, but different doctors have other preferences.

Probenecid (Benemid)

Purpose: To lower blood uric acid.

Indications: For the lowering of blood uric acid in patients who have had acute gout and have not had kidney stones.

Dosage: One 0.5 gram tablet twice daily is standard.

Side effects: These are entirely minimal; very rarely skin rash or stomach upset has been reported.

Special hints: This drug increases the elimination of uric acid by the kidneys. It doesn't interfere in the chemistry of the body very much, since its effects are limited to the kidney. Aspirin will block the effects in the kidneys and should not be used together with probenecid. The drug is well tolerated and has a long and very good safety record. Its cost is only about two-thirds that of allopurinol.

Usually, a doctor will not start probenecid at the time when you are having an attack of acute gouty arthritis, since it may theoretically prolong the attack. It should be started during the interval between attacks in most instances. As it lowers the uric acid, attacks of gout may come even more frequently for the first few months. For this reason, colchicine is usually given as a preventive treatment along with the probenecid; a combination drug including both (Colbenemid) is available. The combination helps to prevent the acute attacks as well as lower the uric acid. Eventually, acute attacks should decrease after treatment with probenecid. Since probenecid increases the amount of uric acid in the urine, it may predispose to kidney stones. We think it is wise for patients to drink a lot of water and even sometimes to use sodium bicarbonate to alkalinize the urine in order to prevent kidney-stone formation.

Many doctors believe that a patient with acute gouty arthritis should have the uric acid in the urine for a 24-hour period measured by the laboratory. Kidney stones can be a complication of too much uric acid in the urine. If the excretion is higher than normal, allopurinol is used to lower the uric acid. If it is normal, probenecid is used. This is quite a rational procedure and can help your doctor select the right drug for you.

Allopurinol (Zyloprim)

Purpose: To reduce uric acid in blood and urine.

Indications: Patients with a history of acute gouty arthritis, uric-acid kidney stone, or both, and who have an elevated 24-hour urine uric acid.

Dosage: Three or four 100 mg tablets per day, or one 300 mg tablet in the morning.

Side effects: These are quite minimal, although more frequent than with probenecid. Up to 5 percent of patients will have a skin rash and a few more will have some stomach upset. The great majority of patients tolerate this drug very well. As a caveat, it must be added that although few serious side effects have been reported in the first fifteen years of our experience with this drug, it profoundly affects body systems and the possibility of unknown side effects still exists. For example, allopurinol can be incorporated into the genetic material and its use does affect some major chemical pathways in the body. Some doctors have identified rare patients with an allergic reaction in the blood vessels due to allopurinol.

Special hints: The main hint for allopurinol is not to use it if you don't need it. The great majority of people receiving allopurinol are just getting it for elevated uric acid without any disease. This is expensive nonsense. Nevertheless, allopurinol represents one of the most important drug developments of this century and it provides a very fundamental aid in the treatment of patients with serious gout problems. Once begun, it should in almost all instances be maintained for life. It is important that allopurinol (or for that matter, probenecid) be taken regularly, even though one feels well. For a patient with gout, the uric acid will decline during treatment with these drugs, but as soon as the drug is stopped, the uric acid will go back to where it was before the drug had been used. Allopurinol is a medical marvel, but falls just a little short of being a miracle.

DRUGS FOR IMMUNE SUPPRESSION

These drugs are experimental. They are hazardous. They are powerful. They are seldom necessary. They are used less now than they were a few years ago.

The immune response helps the body recognize and fight foreign particles and viruses. When it goes wrong, we can have allergy or auto-immune disease. Here, antibodies from the immune system attack the body's own tissues, causing disease. When this response is overexuberant the immunosuppressant drugs can tone it down.

Some of these drugs work by *cytotoxic* action. They kill rapidly dividing cells much like an X-ray beam. Since in some diseases the most rapidly dividing cells are the bad ones, the overall drug effect is good. Others of these drugs antagonize chemical systems inside the cell, such as the purine system or the folate system. From the patient's standpoint, it doesn't make too much difference how they work and they can all be considered about the same. Keep in mind that they are powerful and dangerous.

The major immediate worry is destruction of the bone-marrow cells. All of these drugs can do this if you get too much of them. The bone-marrow cells make platelets that stop bleeding, red cells that carry oxygen, and white cells that fight infection. The bone-marrow cells always are rapidly dividing. Any of these blood-cell types can be suppressed by taking enough of these drugs. Even if there seem to be enough white blood cells, dangerous infections can occur due to reduced effectiveness of the cells.

These infections are often called "opportunistic"; different kinds of germs cause these infections than those that cause infections in healthy people. Frequently we will see *herpes zoster* (shingles). Patients will sometimes get infections with types of fungus that are around all the time but seldom cause disease. Or, a rare bacterial infection can occur. Often these infections are difficult to treat and sometimes hard even to diagnose.

The major long-term worry is cancer. This is a theoretical danger and it may not happen with the treatment of arthritis in humans. These drugs do cause cancer in some laboratory animals. If cancer is caused by these drugs, it happens only after many years. Present evidence suggests that leukemia can occasionally be caused by immunosuppressants.

After considering all these dangers, we really don't know how to compare them to other dangers. Suppose that one patient in one hundred gets cancer, but that ten lives are saved. Suppose that one patient in one hundred gets cancer, but the alternative treatment is prednisone with all of its potential problems. It is possible that these drugs are actually less dangerous than some of the drugs we are currently more comfortable with. Their role is still being carefully considered.

The clearest indications for these drugs, in descending order, are as follows. In Wegener's granulomatosis, previously fatal, these drugs are usually curative and are mandated. They seem helpful in severe polyarteritis. They are probably useful in resistant severe dermatomyositis or polymyositis. They are probably helpful in the severe kidney disease of systemic lupus. They are helpful in psoriatic arthritis and rheumatoid arthritis, but the risks usually outweigh the benefits and here they should be reserved for the most seriously affected patients.

Cyclophosphamide (Cytoxan)

Purpose: For immunosuppression.

Indications: Wegener's granulomatosis, severe systemic lupus erythematosus, polyarteritis, possibly severe rheumatoid arthritis.

Dosage: Usual dose is 100 to 150 mg (two to three tablets) daily.

Side effects: Dosage is usually adjusted so that the white count is maintained in the low normal range. Severe bone-marrow depression can occur and cancer has followed use in laboratory animals. Opportunistic infections can occur. Special side effects of Cytoxan include hair loss, which can be quite extensive but usually reverses after the drug is discontinued, and bladder irritation. The drug is eliminated from the body through the kidneys and the eliminated products can cause blisters on the inside of the bladder. Scarring of the bladder and possibly even cancer of the bladder can result after long-term use. Additionally, there is a decrease in the sperm count and, in women of child-bearing age, there is damage to the eggs which can cause sterility. These effects are reversible at first, but irreversible later. Stomach or intestinal upset is noted by some patients.

Special hints: Cytoxan may be the strongest of the immunosuppressant agents and it is probably the most toxic. Nitrogen mustard, which must be given by vein, is a similar drug with many of the same side effects. It is not used as frequently. The bladder side effects can be minimized by drinking large amounts of water, and all patients taking this drug should endeavor to drink an extra two quarts of liquid each day beyond their usual intake. This dilutes the toxic products in the bladder and minimizes the damage. Don't take this drug at bedtime becaue the concentrated overnight urine will stay in your bladder too long. Use of the drug should be reconsidered by patients planning to have children. Regular blood counts, every one or two weeks to start and no less frequently than once a month later, are required.

Chlorambucil (Leukeran)

Purpose: Immunosuppression.

Indications: Same as cyclophosphamide.

Dosage: One to six 2 mg tablets daily.

Side effects: The same as cyclophosphamide, except hair loss is less frequent and the bladder side effects do not occur.

Special hints: For reasons that are unclear, chlorambucil is not used as frequently as cyclophosphamide, although some investigators prefer it. The bone-marrow suppression is less predictable and can happen a bit more suddenly with chlorambucil according to some investigators. With any of these drugs, regular blood counts, every one to two weeks to begin with and no less frequently than once a month later, are required.

Azathioprine (Imuran); 6-mercaptopurine

Purpose: Immunosuppression, with some anti-inflammatory action.

Indications: Severe systemic lupus erythematosus, severe rheumatoid arthritis, severe psoriatic arthritis, steroid-resistant polymyositis or dermatomyositis.

Dosage: 100 to 150 mg (two or three tablets) daily is the usual.

Side effects: Azathioprine and 6 morcaptopurine (6-MP) are closely related drugs with almost identical actions. Azathioprine is the most frequently used. Side effects include opportunistic infections and possibility of late development of cancer. Gastrointestinal (stomach) distress is occasionally noted. Hair loss is unusual and there appears to be little effect on the sperm or the eggs. There are no bladder problems. Liver damage has been reported. Usually, however, the drug is well tolerated.

Special hints: Regular blood tests are required. Patients taking these drugs should never take allopurinol (Zyloprim), since the combination of drugs can be fatal. After a response is obtained, it is often possible to reduce the dose. Theoretically, this decreases the risk of late side effects. Azathioprine has been shown to slow down the progression of rheumatoid arthritis and is very effective in some patients. Most patients seem not to have any side effects, but we remain concerned about what might happen over the long term.

Methotrexate

Purpose: For immunosuppression.

Indications: Steroid-resistant dermatomyositis or polymyositis, severe psoriatic arthritis.

Dosage: Usually this drug is given intravenously or intramuscularly at intervals of one week to ten days. The dose ranges from 20 to 40 mg each injection. If taken by mouth, it is usually given in three or four doses 8 to 12 hours apart, with a week following during which no drug is given.

Side effects: These include opportunistic infections and the possibility of late development of cancer. The special side effect is damage to the liver. This is particularly a problem if the drug is given by mouth every day; most doctors have discontinued this method of administration. When given by mouth, it is absorbed by the intestine and passes through the liver on the way to general circulation. At this time, liver damage appears to occur. If the drug is given intermittently, there is an opportunity for the liver to heal. If given every day, cirrhosis and severe problems with the liver can result. These problems can still occur with the newer dose schedules, but are much less frequent.

Special hints: Regular blood tests are required as with all of these drugs. Some doctors recommend liver biopsy to be sure that the liver is normal before starting the drug. I personally feel that this procedure is hazardous and is not required if blood liver tests are normal before the drug is started. The blood liver tests should be checked every so often, perhaps at three- or six-month intervals during treatment, and the drug should be stopped if there is any suspicion of difficulty. Since alcohol can damage the liver, alcohol intake should be extremely moderate during a period of methotrexate treatment.

EXPERIMENTAL DRUGS

Don't wait around for a breakthrough. Every day I get calls or letters asking whether there is "anything new for arthritis." Such questions are dangerously misguided. First, delay in proper treatment while waiting for some new remedy may be hazardous. Second, presently available drugs are truly excellent when used in combination with a sound overall program. Third, any new drug will be risky during the first few years, since it takes that long for doctors to get familiar with all of its nuances. Fourth, any new drug powerful enough to be a major help will have severe side effects, some of which will be discovered only many years later. This last point is a prediction, but it has held true for all drugs to date.

It is, of course, interesting to follow developments in pharmaceutical research. Scientific understanding of diseases is mirrored by the treatments doctors prescribe. The expectations of society and the requirements of regulatory bodies are reflected in the process of new-drug introduction. The recent search has been for the perfect aspirin substitute—a nonsteroidal anti-inflammatory agent, safe and effective. This is a huge drug market, and 56 separate drugs are under development. Those drugs already licensed are discussed above; depending on future actions of the FDA, there may be many more.

Many of these other new drugs are presently available in other countries, including Europe and Mexico. These are the drugs people refer to when they say that "better" drugs are available in other countries. Forget these myths. Essentially, the drugs not yet licensed in the United States are the same as the anti-inflammatory agents already licensed here; the best drugs have been rushed fastest to our market to capture the largest market share. Virtually all of these agents have been developed in the United States and are only licensed in foreign countries because licensing is less of a hassle there. As we learn more about the nonsteroidal agents, we will probably find that some are a little better than others under certain circumstances. But no major breakthrough is in sight.

In a slightly different category is development of an oral gold compound. Gold must now be given by injection, weekly, and has severe side effects. Now a tablet that can be taken orally has been developed which appears to give good levels of the gold salt in the blood. Additionally, it may be less toxic and quicker acting. This is not a breakthrough, but might be a major convenience for some patients.

I must venture a negative comment about DMSO. Periodically, the press runs stories about DMSO as an arthritis treatment, usually alleging deliberate suppression of research by the government. A number of people apparently feel that the government is suppressing a cure for arthritis. In some areas, a black market in DMSO, similar to that of Laetrile for cancer, has sprung up. Another strange idiocy. It is true that research was nearly stopped because of toxicity to laboratory animals and fear by the government that human subjects would be exposed to undue risk. This decision may have been wrong and many of us would like to have seen the early research studies completed. I observed some early research studies with DSMO when such investigation was legal. It was a very unimpressive drug! It is an interesting chemical that appeared to have no effect by itself but could carry corticosteroid medication through the skin. Although the steroids could reduce inflammation, they could also damage the skin, and the responses were only for the very short term. Of all of the drugs I have studied as arthritis treatments, DMSO is perhaps the least promising. Certainly its unavailability is no great loss.

Two drugs representing new approaches to arthritis treatment are under development at this time. Levamisole is an immunostimulant. It works in reverse to the immunosuppressants and it is not clear why it should be useful in diseases such as rheumatoid arthritis. Still, some investigators have reported good results, while other investigators have not. Some levamisole investigators have found white-cell depression to be a serious side effect and are worried about the drug's safety. But it does represent a new approach about which we may hear more. Frentizole is an immunosuppressant medication that is not cytotoxic and appears free of some major side effects of present agents. It has seemed as powerful as cyclophosphamide in some tests. Still, its development is in the very early stages and many problems may not yet have been uncovered.

There are many drugs under development that have not been discussed here. These include new drugs for reduction of the uric acid and for prevention of crystal arthritis, short-acting corticosteroid preparations that might be less toxic, combinations of several ingredients, and so forth. A prominent medical spokesman, Dr. Lewis Thomas, would probably say that these represent "half-way technology." Dr. Thomas has pointed out that when we don't know how to tackle a problem, we invent an imperfect solution that costs a lot more money. The new-drug programs for arthritis fall into this category.

There is unlikely to be any "magic" in the new drugs developed over the next few years. Improvement and refinements, yes, but magic, no. Excellent treatment of arthritis is available through the principles outlined in this book. Both arthritis and deformity can be prevented by sound use of present medicines and surgery, together with your hard work. This will result in a good outcome for your arthritis. Get on with it.

What About Surgery?

Surgery can relieve pain, restore function, and return a patient to employment. Its potential for repair of a damaged joint increases year by year. But surgery is expensive and painful, is associated with a long recovery period, keeps you away from activities during the period of convalescence, and may not be successful. The joint might be worse afterward. Surgery can even kill you or paralyze you, although this is rare. The decision for surgery is one that you will make with your doctor. It's a major step and you want to make the right decision. Here are some guidelines to help you sort out the issues.

GENERAL RULES

Surgery for Arthritis is Seldom Urgent

With only a few exceptions, a delay of days, weeks, or even months makes relatively little difference with surgery for arthritis. If the operation is successful, you will have delayed the good result; if the operation is unsuccessful, you will have delayed the pain and expense by waiting. You have plenty of time for a second opinion, or a third. You can watch your condition to see if it will go away by itself or perhaps stabilize at an acceptable level. So, take your time. Rare exceptions to this rule involve bone conditions causing nerve pressure, a bacterial infection in the bone or joint, or a rupture of the tendons.

Not All Surgeons Are Equal

Generally, you will want an orthopedic or hand surgeon to perform any operations on your joints that may be required. You will also want a surgeon who does a lot of joint operations and is up-to-date on the latest techniques. Surgery is a rapidly changing field and familiarity with the most recent advances leads to better results. A surgeon who performs the operation only once or twice a year is not likely to have the same level of skill as a surgeon who does the operation weekly. As a dividend, you will usually find that the busy joint surgeon is more conservative in his or her recommendation for operation. It's not at all uncommon for a good orthopedic surgeon to indicate quite candidly that the condition for which the operation is being considered is not likely to respond to surgical treatment—and then you will be spared the operation.

Not All Operations Are Equal

The total hip replacement and total knee replacement are very fine operations—almost all patients receive some benefit from them. On the other hand, certain procedures, such as tendon operations on the small joints of the hand or most kinds of back surgery, are far less predictable. Before you decide to have either of the latter two kinds of operation, you will want to find out how good the recommended operation is.

Best Results Are Achieved When Problems Are Localized

Medical treatment is often best for a widespread problem. On the other hand, if the problem is localized, say to a knee, then surgery is likely to be a good, targeted approach to the problem. If a large number of joints are involved, surgery may be impractical. For example, the lower extremity has eight major weight-bearing areas: the two forefeet, the ankle, the knees, and the hips. If any one of these areas is limiting walking, surgery may be a wise move. But if all eight areas are bad, then fixing one is not going to be of particular help. Improvement in one joint without relief to the other seven cannot be translated into function and increased activity. Be realistic. Ask how well you would be if the area of a proposed operation were entirely well. If the answer is, "It wouldn't be much different," then the surgery may not be advisable.

Best Results Are Achieved in Treatment of Large Joints

The joint is a complicated structure and healing after surgery can result in stiffness, particularly if the area of the joint is small. The best surgical procedures repair large joints such as the hip and the knee. Results in these areas are usually predictably good. With the smaller joints, sophisticated repair techniques sometimes don't improve function significantly and should be approached with caution. Usually problems with smaller joints are also problems that involve many joints, which again complicates the surgical approach.

Joint Replacement

This is the newest and probably the most important orthopedic surgical procedure for arthritis. The joint is removed and replaced entirely by an artificial joint. The cartilage is replaced by long-wearing plastics such as Teflon, the bone is replaced by stainless steel, and the artificial joint is embedded in the ends of the bones on either side by a marvelous cement called methyl methacralate. This bone cement has made the new era in joint surgery possible by providing a way to anchor the artificial joint to the bones.

The hip was the first joint to be "replaced." Total hip replacement is a marvelous operation in the hands of an experienced surgeon. Pain is almost totally relieved and function greatly improved. The present artificial hip is estimated to last ten to fifteen years, and newer models are expected to last longer as design problems are overcome. The failure rate is only one or two percent, but these patients may have infections or even have to have the artificial hip removed. It is true that some patients receiving artificial hips have had to have a replacement for the replacement; it is also true that this usually has been satisfactory.

The knee is a complicated hinge joint with a requirement for sideways stability. This has made it more difficult to construct an appropriate replacement joint, since the joint must move freely in the hinge direction but must strongly resist sideways force. The ball-and-socket joint of the hip poses easier engineering problems. Techniques of knee replacement have been greatly refined over the last several years.

Ankle replacements remain experimental, as do shoulder replacements. Operations to replace the small joints of the fingers are widely practiced, but the outcome has not been uniformly satisfactory. One of the problems with present operations for the small joints of the hands is that appearance may be considerably improved by the straightening of deformed fingers, but the ability to use the hand may not be greatly changed.

Synovectomy

Removal of inflamed synovium is termed a *synovectomy*. This popular operation results in a reduction of the swelling of synovitis and presumably less enzymatic damage to the joint because the inflamed tissue mass has been reduced. Unfortunately, joint stiffness is often experienced after the synovectomy and the inflamed tissue frequently grows back. There has been a long-standing argument about whether synovectomy should be done early or late in rheumatoid arthritis, with some doctors still holding each extreme position. In other words, the effects of synovectomy are not so dramatic that people can't argue about them. There should be a special reason for this operation, such as worsening of a single joint when all other joints are in control or the hope of avoiding the use of a dangerous drug.

Resections

Some older operations sound a bit bizarre and this is the case with resection procedures. Here, bones are just cut away and removed. This sounds like it wouldn't be very helpful, but often the opposite is true. Resection of the metatarsal heads in the forefoot, for example, can relieve pain and restore the ability to walk. Similar operations may be done in the distal ulna, the bone on the outside of the wrist. Or, bunions and other protuberances can be removed. While this surgery is not elegant in concept, it can be very useful.

Fusions

An operation to unite two bones is termed a *fusion*. Such operations are useful to stabilize joints; the fusion provides a platform for movement and prevents pain in the fused area. The wrist and ankle are the joints where this procedure is most frequently used; fusion of the back is also performed on occasion. A successful fusion, limiting all motion, stops pain. In the area that is fused, flexibility is lost. Usually, a fusion places additional strain on nearby joints that are called on to take over the flexibility functions. Fusion doesn't always work and nonunion can occur. These operations are useful, however, every now and then.

Back Surgery

A discussion about indications for back surgery is beyond the scope of this chapter. Most patients know from talking with friends that unsuccessful back surgery is common. In most cases, the doctor was not very enthusiastic about performing this surgery but the continuing problems of the patient eventually led doctor and patient to agree on this measure. And it didn't work.

By and large, back surgery is not advisable unless there is evidence of pressure on nerve roots. This may happen with a herniated disk, or with narrowing of the spinal canal, or with back fractures.

A myelogram can demonstrate pressure on the nerves in the spinal cord. Operations in patients with negative myelograms are the least likely to succeed. However, the myelogram itself requires placement of a needle into the spinal canal and the injection of a not-innocuous dye into the space around the spinal cord. It is uncomfortable and there are some side effects. Hence, even considering a myelogram should be reserved for the most serious back problems.

The back is composed of an extraordinarily complex set of muscles, ligaments, and tendons. The injury may be anywhere and is frequently not in the spine; hence, surgery on the spine may not be countering what is wrong. Read the sections on the back in Chapter 2 and in problem 12, Part III. Seek multiple opinions before having a back operation. You want to avoid back surgery if you can, and it's mainly up to you.

There can be nerve pressure out in the limbs. An example is the carpal-tunnel syndrome where there is pressure on the nerve passing over the front of the wrist and pain and tingling in the fingers. This pressure can be effectively eliminated by surgery and surgery should be undertaken if rest and injection do not result in disappearance of the syndrome within a few weeks. Other problems, such as a Morton's neuroma, can also cause peripheral pain. Here, an injury has caused the nerve fibers to grow into a little ball and to transmit pain signals all the time. If this bundle of nerves is removed, the pain is eliminated and a good result obtained. So, while we can't really operate to repair nerves, we can either remove the structures that are pressing on them or remove the area that is sending the abnormal signals.

Cosmetic Surgery

We use the term *cosmetic* here in a disparaging way. Usually, surgery for the joint should be done only to relieve pain or improve function. The appearance of the joint is much less important. Some operations serve mainly to improve appearance. Many patients are later disappointed by such operations. The appearance is less than perfect anyway and the patient somehow had been expecting that the part would work better if it looked better, despite advice to the contrary.

Understanding Those Tests

There are four general rules to remember about tests. First, no test is perfect. Normal people sometimes have abnormal tests and people with arthritis often test normally. Usually these are not laboratory errors but reflect the imperfection of the test. Doctors describe tests by their "sensitivity" and "specificity." No test has perfect sensitivity, meaning that it detects all cases, and perfect specificity, meaning that no normal persons have a positive test.

Second, tests do not establish the diagnosis or treatment. Rather, they confirm the impression of the physician. Any doctor who relies entirely on tests to make decisions is a bad doctor. Your doctor should have a pretty good idea of what is going on with your joints before any tests are performed; the tests will help reduce any remaining uncertainty.

Third, explanations will differ as different doctors try to make difficult concepts understandable. Don't worry if you get two quite different explanations for the same test result. Some explanations may even seem absurd to the literal wordsmith, such as, "There is a little bit of arthritis in your blood"—an obvious contradiction in terms. The doctor in this instance is just trying to explain that a blood test frequently associated with arthritis is positive.

Fourth, in general, too many tests are performed. Don't demand tests or feel slighted if no tests are ordered. Often, the experienced physician will use fewer tests. Tests for diagnosis usually don't need to be repeated after the diagnosis has been made. Tests designed to check for drug side effects or to measure improvement may need to be repeated at regular intervals.

In the discussion that follows, we have usually indicated (in italics) how often a test is required and how frequently, if at all, it should be repeated.

These guidelines should give you a frame of reference for understanding the tests requested for your case.

The discussions are short, nontechnical, and grouped by the type of test. We have listed only the most common. The list will still seem complicated, but any individual should only have a few tests. Read about those that pertain to you.

BLOOD TESTS

Hematocrit (PCV—Packed Cell Volume)

This test, and the closely related hemoglobin test, measures the number of red blood cells. The number of red blood cells will be decreased (anemia) with chronic inflammation, as in rheumatoid arthritis, and the degree of reduction corresponds to the severity of the disease. The number can also be reduced if you are losing blood through your bowel as a result of medications, or if a powerful drug has decreased the production of red cells by the bone marrow. (*Commonly employed test; often repeated frequently.*)

White Blood Count (WBC)

The white blood cells help fight infection. With infection the number is often increased and with some drug reactions the number can be decreased. A *differential white count* will sometimes be used to determine the particular kind of white cells being increased or decreased. (*Commonly employed test; often repeated to test for drug side effects or for the possibility of infection.*)

Platelet Count

The platelets help the blood to clot. If the platelet count is too low, there is a possibility of a bleeding problem. This may occur in lupus and in a few of the other diseases discussed in this book, and several of the drugs used to treat arthritis can, rarely, cause the count to be very low. (*Infrequently required test; repetition frequent if the patient is taking a suspect drug.*)

Sedimentation Rate (ESR, Sed Rate)

This can be a valuable test. It tends to measure the amount of inflammation present; a high sed rate means a lot of inflammation. It can help the doctor distinguish between an inflammatory condition and a noninflammatory one. It can help determine whether the inflammation is increasing or decreasing. The test is an old and very simple one. Blood is allowed to settle in a test tube and the distance that it settles in one hour is the sedimentation rate. If there is no inflammation, the sedimentation rate is usually less than 20 mm per hour. (*Commonly used test; often repeated fairly frequently.*)

BLOOD SERUM CHEMISTRY TESTS

Creatinine

This test measures how well the kidneys excrete waste products. A normal creatinine is less than 1.5 mg%; the creatinine may rise to 10 or even 20 if kidney involvement is extremely severe. This test is generally not needed except in diseases such as lupus or polyarteritis, which may cause kidney disease. *(Infrequently required; sometimes repeated observations are necessary.)*

BLOOD SERUM IMMUNOLOGY TESTS

Latex (Rheumatoid Factor, RF, Rose Test)

Many patients with rheumatoid arthritis have a large amount of *rheumatoid factor* circulating in their blood. These factors are also found in patients with no disease at all and in patients with other diseases, although less frequently than in rheumatoid arthritis. A latex test isn't worth much unless it has a *titer* associated with it. The titer tells how much of the rheumatoid factor is present. Patients with rheumatoid arthritis usually have a titer of 1:160 or greater and normal people usually have lower titers. Some other diseases also can cause high titers. The rheumatoid-factor titer is sometimes used to document improvement, but it isn't terribly useful for this *(Required fairly frequently for diagnosis; repeated infrequently.)*

Antinuclear Antibody Tests (ANA, FANA)

Antinuclear antibodies can be found in normal individuals, particularly with increasing age. However, they are almost always present in patients with lupus and are often found in patients with rheumatoid arthritis or other connective-tissue diseases. If the ANA is negative, a diagnosis of lupus is unlikely. Warning: these tests are often overinterpreted and cause unnecessary concern, because a positive test doesn't necessarily mean disease. A positive test can be caused by drugs or just by the aging process. A high titer increases the chance of lupus or a related disease, and doctors get some additional information from the *pattern of fluorescence. (ANA tests are required infrequently and do not require frequent repeat testing, because values change very slowly.)*

DNA (Anti-DNA, DNA Binding, Farr Test)

Several tests measure antibody to DNA, an important body protein. Antibody to DNA is found almost exclusively in the disease lupus. In lupus, if the amount of DNA antibody rises, the situation is potentially more severe.

(Required in very few patients, essentially only those with lupus, but such patients may require testing as often as monthly.)

ENA (Extractable Nuclear Antibody)

This test measures an antibody to an antigen that is found in connective-tissue diseases and is characteristic of an unusual syndrome called MCTD or "mixed connective-tissue disease," which combines features of myositis, lupus, and scleroderma described earlier. When this syndrome is present, a very high titer to the ENA is usually found, perhaps as high as 1:100,000 or 1:1,000,000. *(Infrequently required; since it changes only very slowly, repeat tests are seldom required.)*

Complement (C-3, C-4, B-1-C Protein)

The complement proteins tend to be reduced when lupus is active. The normal and abnormal values vary depending on the laboratory and the particular technique used. *(Required in few patients, essentially only those patients with lupus, but may then be repeated periodically.)*

TISSUE-TYPING TESTS

B-27 (HLA-B27)

Tissue-typing tests originally were developed to improve the results in organ transplantation, such as of the kidneys or heart. As a by-product, the fascinating relationship between the B-27 tissue type and attachment arthritis was discovered. This arthritis runs in families and is found in some of those family members who have the B-27 gene. The gene is transmitted by either the father or mother, and approximately one-half of the children will have the gene. In some instances, this test can help in the diagnosis of arthritis. The tissue type is similar to the familiar blood type, but is done by typing the white cells rather than the red cells. *(Infrequently required, and only when there is suspicion of an attachment arthritis; need not be repeated, since it does not change.)*

URINE TESTS

Urinalysis

This is actually a number of tests. In the area of arthritis, we look for red blood cells, protein, or casts in the urine. These findings suggest nephritis and are sometimes encountered in lupus or arteritis. In addition, drugs such as gold and penicillamine can cause protein loss through the urine. Normal urine has very few red blood cells, no urine protein, and no casts.

(Frequently employed; may be repeated in diseases where kidney involve-
ment is possible or with a drug that might cause kidney damage.)

139
Biopsies

24-Hour Urine Tests (24-Hour Protein; 24-Hour Creatinine Clearance)

These tests determine how much of a particular compound is excreted in 24 hours. So, all urine excreted in a full day is collected. This can give a more accurate estimate of the amount of protein leakage, and the *creatinine clearance* can give an accurate measure of kidney function. Creatinine is a chemical compound found in blood urine, and muscle. The creatinine clearance is calculated from the blood-creatinine value and the 24-hour urine creatinine. This is a cumbersome way to measure kidney function, but is preferred by some doctors to the serum-creatinine value alone. *(The 24-hour protein test will be used only when a routine urinalysis shows that there is some protein leakage. The 24-hour creatinine clearance may be obtained as a "baseline" in a disease where kidney disease is possible, and may be followed serially.)*

BIOPSIES

Skin Biopsy

A small piece of skin may be removed and examined under the microscope to confirm a diagnosis of scleroderma or of some forms of arteritis. It may be used to confirm a diagnosis of lupus, psoriasis, or other skin conditions. The procedure is virtually painless and leaves a small scar. It is done under local anethesia, very quickly, and does not require hospitalization. *(Usually does not need to be repeated.)*

Kidney Biopsy (Renal Biopsy)

This procedure is more hazardous than the skin biopsy. Through a needle inserted in the back, a small core of kidney tissue is removed and examined under the microscope. Complications, particularly bleeding, can occur; blood transfusions are required after one to three percent of kidney biopsies. Death has resulted, but this is exceedingly rare. Very rarely, the bleeding may require removal of the kidney. There is controversy about how frequently these tests should be performed. I use them very rarely, some other doctors use them more frequently.

Muscle Biopsy

Biopsy of the muscle is a safe and easy procedure resulting in a small scar; it is little more difficult than a skin biopsy. Sometimes skin and muscle biopsies are done together. The muscle biopsy finds its greatest value in the diagnosis of polymyositis or dermatomyositis or in the documentation of inflammation in the arteries (arteritis).

Temporal Artery Biopsy

In this biopsy, a piece of the artery that runs across the temple is removed. One or both temporal arteries may be biopsied. This biopsy is simple and has few complications. It can be useful in the diagnosis of giant-cell (temporal) arteritis and is sometimes performed in polymyalgia rheumatica (PMR). It sounds like a major procedure to cut out a piece of an artery, but the scalp is so well supplied with blood vessels that you really don't need this one. Some patients who have headaches related to temporal artery inflammation actually get relief from their headaches after the biopsy. This biopsy is used only when there is a suspicion of giant-cell arteritis, temporal arteritis, or polymyalgia rheumatica (PMR).

JOINT-FLUID TESTS

A needle can be placed into a joint in order to remove joint fluid for laboratory analysis. The procedure is generally easy, particularly in the knee, does not require hospitalization, and has very few complications (infection is the most common). Complications are slightly higher if a substance is injected into the joint.

This test seems like such a direct way to get information about arthritis that it is disappointing that it isn't of more use. It is required if the doctor suspects infection in the joint space, since the particular bacteria can be cultured and identified. It is highly useful if crystal arthritis is suspected and a firm diagnosis has not been made, because identification of the crystals absolutely proves that a crystal arthritis is present. (Occasionally, a crystal arthritis will be present, but the crystals will not be seen.) Examination of the joint fluid can assist in determining whether the arthritis is extremely inflammatory or not. However, the tests performed on the fluid, including cell counts, joint-fluid sugar level, mucin clot tests, and protein measurement, do not absolutely distinguish one kind of arthritis from another except with positive identification of crystals or germs.

X-RAYS

In general, be cautious about X-rays; you are probably aware of the hazards of radiation exposure. There is a popular impression that X-rays give doctors much more information than they actually do. Only the bony structures are well seen on X-rays; problems that affect "soft" tissues of the body don't really show up. The doctor can often tell by examination exactly what would be revealed by an X-ray, so the X-ray wouldn't contribute anything. Further, changes to bone usually take several years to develop; if the arthritis hasn't persisted too long, there is a strong likelihood that the X-ray examination will be normal. The critical question in any test that involves expense or hazard is whether it will add any information to that which is already known. X-rays too often are requested by patients and many patients seem disappointed if the doctor does not recommend X-rays.

Hand X-Rays

These X-rays may be obtained every couple of years in rheumatoid and some other forms of arthritis to determine the rate of bony destruction, if any. Severe rheumatoid arthritis causes small holes near the ends of the bones and the increase in extent of these erosions is a measure of disease progression. Psoriatic arthritis shows a strange "whittled" appearance in some cases and osteoarthritis shows narrowing of the joint spaces and development of bone spurs.

Sacroiliac X-Rays

X-rays of the sacroiliac joints are important in ankylosing spondylitis. The diagnosis is defined to include damage to the sacroiliac joints. Without this X-ray, the diagnosis cannot be made. The X-ray examination of the sacroiliac joints is more important than the B-27 test or other findings that suggest ankylosing spondylitis. After a year or so of ankylosing spondylitis the margins of the sacroiliac joints begin to blur and the bone becomes a bit more dense near the joint. Later, the joint space narrows. In advanced disease the joint entirely disappears, with bone replacing what used to be the sacroiliac joint. These joints are seldom involved in ordinary low back syndromes or in other kinds of arthritis. So, these X-rays are usually required only in patients with suspected attachment arthritis. I prefer to get a single X-ray film of the pelvis to inspect the sacroiliac joints, because I am able to see a little bit of the hip joints and the lower spine as well. Some other doctors prefer to get special angled pictures of the sacroiliac joints themselves.

Cervical Spine (C-Spine) X-Rays

Neck views are frequently requested for osteoarthritis, particularly if pain from the neck extends into the arms or there is weakness in the hands. The doctor is looking for narrowing of the holes through which the nerves pass and for narrowing of the disks. Unfortunately, the X-rays can be pretty confusing. Many patients with narrowed holes for the nerves have no problem whatsoever; others with problems have relatively normal X-rays. Rheumatoid arthritis can affect the upper one or two vertebrae in the spine, just at the base of the skull, and juvenile arthritis also can affect the neck.

Lumbar Spine (L-Spine) X-Rays

Low back syndromes, unless they have been recurrent or are associated with nerve symptoms, don't really require an X-ray. If a disk problem is suspected, some information may be obtained by a plain X-ray, although, like the cervical spine, the results can be confusing. Many patients have symptoms without much abnormality and other patients have a lot of abnormality without any symptoms. The myelogram, a more extensive X-ray in which dye is injected into the spinal canal, is more accurate in identifying nerve pressure. In attachment arthritis, the lumbar spine can be involved and X-rays can depict the degree of involvement. This X-ray is greatly overused and is often done only because patients (or lawyers) seem to expect it.

Areas of Pain and Discomfort

Almost any part of the body can be X-rayed. Calcium deposits may be located in the shoulder, arthritis in the feet may be investigated, and problems in the knees, hips, or other joints can be examined. It doesn't usually make much sense to X-ray areas that aren't painful, since they are usually normal. And, if the pain hasn't been present for very long, a normal X-ray is likely. Finally, treatment for most local conditions, such as tennis elbow, isn't likely to be improved by an X-ray. A good practice is to let your doctor suggest the X-ray—don't bring up the subject yourself.

7

Duck That Quack

Where there are persons who consider themselves "victims," there are apt to be others who consider themselves "predators." Over one-half of persons with significant arthritis participate as victims in one or another confidence game at some point. Usually the person who solicits quack treatments has seen a physician first, so to some extent the existence of quackery reflects a failure of traditional medicine to set proper expectations and to deliver hope. When I ask a patient why he or she went to some improbable healer, the answer is usually, "The doctors didn't seem to be able to do anything." People don't like to have a chronic disease, don't like to be told that they have to do some of the work toward a cure, and don't like to learn that the answer is not simple. The trademark of the false healer is a simple, easy, and exclusive cure.

WHAT DO YOU HAVE TO LOSE?

What's the harm? If a quack treatment isn't dangerous, why not give it a try? (And it usually isn't dangerous, with a few notable exceptions described below. For obvious reasons, a quack treatment that directly harms people won't last long.) What do you have to lose from the quack? More than you think, but you have to consider the issues carefully to understand all that has been lost. Among the losses are: money, courage, will, patience, confidence, dignity, function, life.

Money is the most obvious loss to quackery and has been estimated at several hundred million dollars a year in the United States. The cost can range from a few dollars for a quack book or a copper bracelet to many thousands of dollars for fraudulent injections or heavily promoted spa treatments. Almost all arthritis frauds make a lot of visible money for somebody, be it an author, a practitioner, or an institution. This is your money. Since others would quickly adopt any treatment that truly helped a lot of people, a gimmick being used by only one or two practitioners is highly suspect.

Courage and will are precious attributes for the patient with arthritis, and they are eroded by the disillusionment experienced after a false cure fails. The patience of the arthritis patient may be sorely tried by valid treatments—he or she certainly doesn't need additional quack-treatment failures. Confidence is a closely related attribute. If you have confidence in your doctor you will do better than if you don't. A pattern of rejection of any suggestion made by the doctor is often a vicious aftermath of quack treatment. These losses have to do with loss of the spirit.

Dignity is another profound loss. You were taken in. You were the mark. Somebody manipulated you. You were taken advantage of. You were gullible, stupid, suckered, ripped-off. Your pride, integrity, and autonomy are shaken. Perhaps you overcompensate by clinging to a pathetic belief in the fraud even after it fails. You rationalize. Trying to salvage your dignity, you may even tell your friends that it worked. Not much harm in arthritis fraud, is there?

Displacement of sound treatment by a fraudulent treatment can result in disability or death. Even if you tell yourself that the quack treatment will be in addition to sound treatment, this is unlikely to hold true. Confidence in the sound treatment is apt to be undermined by the self-promotion of the quack treatment. For example, one widely distributed quack book tells patients not to take gold treatments; it's hard to know how much damage has been done by this advice, but it must be considerable. A patient of mine stopped good treatment for her systemic lupus after quack advice, and the chain of events that followed led to the loss of function of both her kidneys and one eye.

Direct side effects of quack treatments can lead to death. Prednisone and phenylbutazone given by quack promoters have caused fatalities and major complications. Mexican-border clinics have been the source of many of these prescriptions.

The terms *quack* and *fraud* are used in this chapter to refer to treatments that lack a rationale acceptable to scientific consensus and that are not supported by acceptable evidence for effectiveness. In other words, there is no reason to think they should work and no evidence that they do. By use of these strong words, I do not mean to imply that all quack practitioners have self-serving, malicious intentions; some sincerely believe in their treatments. I also do not intend to ascribe omniscience to the present scientific consensus, which is likely to be in error in a variety of ways we do not yet suspect.

However, I follow about 2,000 patients with various forms of arthritis. About 20 percent, to my knowledge, have seen a quack at some point. A few have reported some degree of temporary improvement; the rest have bitterly described failure. I have never seen a beneficial response from such treatment that wasn't to be expected without the treatment. I have personally observed repeated treatment failures and adverse complications.

THE WRITTEN WORD AS QUACKERY

Supermarkets and newstands carry publications that remain technically short of pure fantasy but distort minor therapeutic advances into dramatic curative breakthroughs. There usually is some tenuous basis for the story and sometimes the authorities cited are actually experts of considerable stature. The "arthritis cure" headline is repeated every four to six months, always with a different cure.

Usually, the headlines are more misleading than the content of the article, but all tricks are used. The sensational part is on the front page; only after purchasing the paper do you turn to the far less sensational information on the inside. Old information is treated as new, slight changes are described as dramatic, and quotations are taken out of context. The articles are sensational, simplistic, quick, and easy. They tell you what you want to believe. Every such issue wastes a lot of doctor time and patient concern by necessitating discussion and explanation of the nonissues raised.

Quack books may employ a similar sales tactic. The title is likely to contain the words "safe," "easy," "proven," or "cure." There is generally a single, rather thin gimmick purported to be the author's discovery after years of "research"; the rest of the book is padding around the gimmick. There may be an M.D. or D.O. as author, or there may be a preface by an M.D. or a D.O. The treatment is "proved effective" on the basis of letters received, and portions of letters are sometimes included in the text. If there is any reference to the scientific medical literature, most references are to the 1920–1950 period.

I have reviewed every such book that I could find. The gimmicks employed include cod-liver oil, eating foods in the right order, frequent enemas, fish diets, vinegar and honey diets, vitamin C, vitamin D, vitamin E, vitamin A, and others. If the subject were not so serious, the explanations developed would be amusing. One suggests, for example, that cod-liver oil will "oil" the joints. Such theories are an insult to the intelligence of the most naive reader. Avoid all books with the formula described above. Look for favorable mention by the Arthritis Foundation, by the National Institutes of Health, or by major universities.

SOME WELL-PUBLICIZED "CURES"

Flu shots. Yep, three flu shots cure arthritis and you can get them in California for only $400. These clever doctors are entirely legal and even have you sign a paper saying that you were not told the shots would cure your arthritis.

Bee stings. Bee-venom desensitization cures arthritis according to several doctors; for a fee, they will give you a series of injections. This is a carry-over from a treatment popular many years ago—before it was discarded as worthless.

Mexican-border-clinic pills. Several "clinics" exist in Mexican border towns which attract considerable United States money. This is probably the most malignant arthritis fraud being perpetrated at the present time. These pills are dangerous and have killed people. The dispensers lie about the content of the pills. The pills contain a corticosteroid and sometimes other dangerous medications like phenylbutazone, but this is denied by the dispenser even when directly questioned. I have had pills from these clinics analyzed on no less than twelve separate occasions, and each time the analysis found a cortisonelike drug. These pills give days of relief and years of consequences.

Elsewhere in Mexico there are fine physicians of high principle who are genuinely expert in the management of patients with rheumatic diseases. The indictment above is not in any way reflective of medical care in Mexico but rather of specific fraudulent clinics operating along the United States-Mexico border.

Copper bracelets. Just kind of silly.

Acupuncture. The acupuncture fad arrived at a time when political barriers against exchange with China were decreasing. In our haste to welcome Chinese wisdom back into the world community, we overlooked some rather basic observations. Acupuncture has a long and noble history in China and has been developed for uses that are alien to our Western appreciation. For example, acupuncture is used to some extent as anesthesia for surgical operations.

However, acupuncture is *not* used for the treatment of rheumatoid arthritis in China and is felt by Chinese acupuncturists to be ineffective for this purpose. It is used in China for treatment of certain local conditions. In our haste to accept, we invented uses that had long since been discarded by the societies we were trying to accept. Several good scientific studies were done in the United States to determine the usefulness of acupuncture for rheumatoid arthritis and osteoarthritis, particularly of the knees. The studies showed no effect on the arthritis, although one study showed a slight decrease in pain, rather less than with aspirin.

Acupressure. An ingenious, timely, novel, and worthless extrapolation of acupuncture.

And then there is Madison Avenue.

- "More of the pain reliever doctors recommend most." (Translation: simple aspirin, overpriced.)

- "Extra-strength formula." (Translation: more overpriced aspirin.)

- "As much pain relief as you can get without a doctor's prescription." (Translation: overpriced aspirin or acetominophen.)

Such attempts to deceive the public are deserving of contempt. Since the claims are technically factual, the advertising is apparently legal. Perhaps we need a sales boycott by consumers. Anacin, Excedrin, and Empirin are among the best-selling and most heavily advertised brands. There is no medical reason of which I am aware why you should ever buy any of these heavily advertised products for arthritis. Less expensive products with the same ingredients will save you money—and you will be taking a stand for honesty in product promotion.

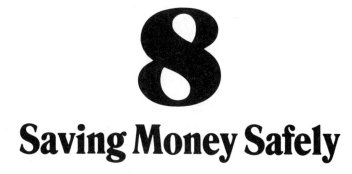

Saving Money Safely

Money is money. You don't want to let the notion "nothing is too much for my health" fool you into blindly purchasing goods or services that could equally well be purchased for substantially less. Nor do you want "insurance will cover it" to keep you from being as careful a consumer as you are with your other purchases. We all pay insurance premiums and we all have the obligation to keep them as low for ourselves as we can. Your taxes, which pay a big chunk of medical expenses, are related to the medical bills you run up. Regardless of who pays the bill now, *you* pay it over the long term.

Health is indeed more important than money. This chapter is about saving money without sacrificing health—hence the title, "Saving Money Safely." The suggestions offered in this chapter can save you 50 percent or more on the costs incurred by your arthritis. Only a few of these suggestions may be applicable to you or your family in an individual case, but use the ones that apply, after checking with your doctor.

SAVING MONEY ON MEDICATIONS

Take as few different medications as possible. "Polypharmacy" is usually an indication of less than optimal medical care. Ask the doctor if all of the medications are necessary. Problems with multiple medications include increased likelihood of side effects from at least one, potential ill effects from the chemical interactions between the different drugs, and the small amount of benefit that is likely to accrue. If three drugs don't fix you up, four are very unlikely to do the trick. The good patient looks for substitution of one medication for another if a program is not going well rather than addition of one drug to another.

Take medication as directed. "Saving pills" is false economy and may impair your health and ultimately be more costly. Some pills can be taken as you feel you need them; many must be taken very regularly. Check with your doctor. If you don't follow instructions, your doctor may not be able to evaluate correctly the cause of your problem and the effectiveness of prescribed medication. As a consequence, your health may be adversely affected.

Throw out old medications. Anything over three years old should go—earlier if it is past the expiration date on the package. Saving old medications is false economy.

Use *generic* medications whenever possible. These are medicines sold by their chemical name rather than the brand name, and they are not protected by patent. So, competitive prices make them less expensive. Ask your doctor if a generic medication is possible. For example, prednisone (a generic drug) costs only one-tenth to one twentieth as much as Medrol, Decadron, Aristocort, and other steroids bought by brand name. Yet prednisone is the best understood of all of these drugs. Phenylbutazone is another drug available in generic prescription. Soon, indomethacin will be available in generic formulation.

Don't request "new" drugs. Usually your expectations for such drugs are unrealistically high and these agents are always expensive. Your doctor will suggest a new drug to you if it seems to have particular promise.

Avoid unnecessary drugs. Know the purpose of each and make sure it makes sense. For example, allopurinol or probenecid are most frequently prescribed for asymptomatic hyperuricemia, a minor laboratory abnormality that isn't even a disease. Patients may spend $170 a year for life as a result of such unnecessary prescriptions. Other situations in which drugs might be unnecessary are long-term treatment for local conditions or treatment during asymptomatic periods. Check with your doctor as to whether the medication need be continued.

Minimize the use of painkillers. Darvon, Talwin, codeine, Percodan, Empirin #3, Tylenol #3, and so forth have a very limited role in treatment of arthritis. Avoid these when possible and take as few as possible if you take any at all.

Minimize the use of tranquilizers and mood drugs. Amphetamines, Dexamyl, Valium, Librium, Dalmane, and a variety of other best-selling agents that lift you up, put you down, or keep you asleep have a very limited role in the management of arthritis. Avoid such drugs whenever possible and take as few as possible.

Avoid combination drugs. You seldom need all of the elements of a combination drug, just as you don't usually need many separate drugs. In the combination drug, the proportion of the drugs is fixed and flexibility is lost. You pay for the unneeded ingredients in increased costs and side effects.

Avoid heavily advertised drugs. Excedrin, Anacin, Empirin, Ascriptin, and Arthritis Pain Formula, among others, have no advantage and some disadvantages over standard USP preparations. They may cost five to ten times as much. There is no reason ever to buy any of these drugs for your arthritis.

Watch out for injections. By and large, injections of painkillers or cortisone into joints or ligaments should be performed rather sparingly. Usually, simpler things should be tried first, and injection into a painful area shouldn't be repeated more than a few times. It is all right to question your doctor if too many injections are suggested. Sometimes they are needed, often not.

SAVING MONEY ON LABORATORY TESTS

Don't ask for trouble by requesting tests, expecting them, or being disappointed if none are ordered. The best doctors are very selective in the ordering of tests. Patient requests are a major reason for performance of some very doubtful procedures. You can keep the pressure off.

Keep records of previous tests and bring the results to your doctor. Avoid the expensive repetition of laboratory work that has already been performed. A major reason for ordering laboratory tests is simply that records have been lost or are unavailable.

Some laboratory tests should be repeated periodically throughout an illness; some should not. Check Chapter 6 to get some feeling for how often a particular test should be ordered. Don't repeat tests that have value only the first time.

Laboratory test schedules can often be simplified. For example, if you are having tests of blood and urine to detect toxicity from gold injections, there are several acceptable means for the doctor to check for toxicity. The simplest ones cost about $300 for a 20-week initial course of gold, just for the laboratory testing. This is costly enough, but the more complicated schedules offer no additional safety and cost about $800. Ask your doctor to check on this.

Can you do it yourself? Some laboratory tests, such as urinalysis, can be performed at home without special training or much expense. Patients with diabetes do it all the time by testing the urine with a piece of test paper that turns color to indicate the contents of the urine. If your urine is being checked regularly to monitor for drug side effects, you may want to check it yourself at home and keep a chart to bring to the doctor.

Can you have it done closer to home? Transportation and your time are hidden costs involved in laboratory testing. If you can find a good laboratory with a more convenient location you may be able to save significant amounts of time and money. Laboratories will release results to you if so instructed by your physician or the results can be mailed directly to the doctor.

SAVING MONEY ON X-RAYS

Again, don't ask for trouble. Patient requests are a major reason for performance of X-rays that have limited medical value. X-rays involve radiation, although the amount is small; they also cost money and this amount is often not small. Let the doctor suggest X-rays if necessary.

One X-ray or several? For X-rays of the hands, feet, and the sacroiliac joints, often one picture is as useful as several different views. The cost differential is considerable. Check with the doctor to see if several views are required and, if not, request the simpler procedure. Less radiation and less cost are both desirable.

Be especially careful with major X-rays—the upper GI (gastrointestinal) series, the barium enema, the arteriogram, and so forth. These are expensive, uncomfortable procedures, they take a good bit of time, and they may, in rare instances, cause you some difficulty. They aren't required very often for arthritis and you ought to be sure that you understand the need for them if they are ordered.

Repeat X-rays are not needed very often. Usually the interval should be at least one year between X-ray examinations and often five years is the more appropriate interval. If infection is suspected, the doctor may need X-rays more frequently, but make sure you understand the need for frequent repeat X-rays.

Get your previous X-rays. It takes a little bit of work to pry your old X-rays out of the file room where they are stored in order to take them to a new health facility. But it is well worth the hassle. You don't want X-rays repeated just because the old ones aren't readily available.

Question the *skeletal* survey. It is very easy for the doctor to order a skeletal survey, which is an X-ray of essentially all of the bones of the body. In arthritis, only certain areas of the body will be of real interest on the X-ray. The extra expense and radiation from the additional X-ray films can be safely avoided. On the other hand, there are instances in which the survey may be less costly than a bunch of separate X-rays. So, question.

Question the baseline X-ray. Sometimes X-rays are obtained simply as a benchmark for future X-ray comparison. "Just in case" is often not a good enough reason for the expense and radiation of X-rays. If you are trying to save a few dollars, avoiding baseline X-rays is a good way to cut costs. Doctors differ on this point, but I almost never find the need for a baseline X-ray.

SAVING MONEY ON DOCTOR VISITS

Get a doctor—one doctor, in whom you have confidence. If you and your doctor don't get along, change doctors, but change early rather than often. Doctor shopping and doctor switching waste time, money, and health.

Don't go to the doctor too soon. Refer to the chart in Chapter 1 and those following in Part III for instructions about the appropriate interval between initial concern and a visit to the doctor.

Don't go too often. Work out the needed frequency of visitation with your physician. Consider this: If you go to the doctor every two weeks, it costs twice as much as it does to go every four weeks. Even less expensive may be an arrangement where you call for an appointment if a problem needs attention. Decisions about how often to see a patient are often made casually without much thought about what the exact interval should be. There is often lots of room for discussion, so ask your doctor. In some locations a nurse practitioner can help with routine problems at less cost.

Duck the quack. Chapter 7 suggests ways to avoid funneling your money into the pockets of those waiting to exploit you.

Ask for a second opinion. If there is a big decision you aren't sure of, check it out. It costs a little extra to be certain, but you may be able to avoid the procedure altogether. This is often important for surgical decisions and sometimes for large medical decisions, such as institution of treatment with gold salts, immunosuppressants, or penicillamine.

Question referrals you don't understand. If your doctor is referring you too frequently, you may be better off with a specialist who knows how to manage your problems. If too many consultations and referrals are needed, your care can become expensive and fragmented. A "Rheumatologist" is also a specialist in Internal Medicine and usually can help with your general medical problems as well.

SAVING MONEY ON HOSPITALS

Don't go into the hospital unless it is essential. There are relatively few reasons for hospitalization of the patient with arthritis. Among the doubtful indications are hospitalization for uncomplicated low back syndromes, for biopsy procedures, because of a bad home situation, or for a series of tests. Usually another less expensive, less time consuming, and equally good for you solution can be found in such circumstances. If you do enter the hospital for a "borderline" reason, the insurance company may refuse to pay after you have already run up a large bill. We have seen some really tragic instances of this problem. If you work effectively with your doctor on your home program, you usually should do well and not require hospitalization.

Look for facilities at lower cost. Increasingly, hospitals offer a range of services for patients with different kinds of problems. The intensive-care unit may now cost $800 per day, but facilities where you do some self-care at much lower costs may be available. You might want to consider them.

Go home soon. Hospitalizations often drag along beyond "MHB" —maximal hospital benefit. Often this is because the patient exerts pressure on the physician to stay in the hospital a few extra days. This is not a healthy habit for you; as soon as you are able, go home.

Have procedures scheduled before admission. Preadmission testing is possible in many hospitals and can decrease the stay by a day or more. If you have surgery, go into the hospital for the minimum time required before the procedure is scheduled.

Avoid hospitalization during a weekend. The hospital slows down over the weekend; the laboratory and other facilities are not staffed as completely. If a weekend intervenes in your hospitalization, it may result in a couple of wasted days.

Understand and question. This is really the point of all the suggestions above. The world is changing. Good doctors and good clinics will understand your financial questions. As an intelligent consumer, you have the right to agree or disagree with those things that are being done for you and to you. Pose your questions thoughtfully and work out solutions that are comfortable for both you and the doctor. Arthritis care can be very expensive. Your problem may last many months or even many years. It may involve expenses in all of the areas discussed above and it may impact your ability to remain employed. Protection of your financial security is an essential element of good medical treatment. Personal bankruptcy is not conducive to improving health. The impact of nonmedical factors, such as personal finances, on medical outcome is increasingly recognized. The good physician will be sympathetic and helpful with your financial problems.

9
Preventing Arthritis

Perhaps you don't have arthritis (yet). Or your family and friends see your arthritis and want to know what they can do to protect themselves. Just as it is important to take preventive measures against heart disease and cancer, it is important to prevent problems with the bones, joints, and muscles. As you get older, you need reserve strength in your heart muscle. You also need reserve strength in your muscles and joints. The techniques for preventing arthritis are simple but not easy. You have to work at them. There is a big bonus, however. By maintaining a life-style healthy for arthritis, you also protect your heart, and the measures you need to protect against arthritis will make you feel better, will give you more energy, and will extend your life. So, there are rewards for the hard work. The three major things you need to do are: keep fit, control your weight, and protect your joints.

KEEP FIT

Exercise has many benefits for us. First, our bones increase in strength —use of our bones causes the calcium content to increase and the trusses that support our weight to thicken. Ligaments tighten and become thicker with use, providing better support for the joint structures. Cartilage is nourished by motion of the joint, which brings oxygen into the cartilage and takes the waste products out. For arthritis prevention you need strong bones, strong supporting ligaments, and healthy cartilage. Exercise is the way to get these.

Exercise for arthritis prevention must be a regular part of your life. It should be repeated daily. Your exercise program should be expanded only

155

very slowly from your beginning level. Plan to maintain your healthy habits for the rest of your life. There is no hurry. Slow and steady does it. Great strength doesn't help. Weight lifting, push-ups, pull-ups, and so forth are not of benefit. Repetitious but less strenuous activities such as walking, biking, and swimming are superb. The muscles gain tone, the bones gain strength, and the ligaments gain both flexibility and strength. Start with walking, bicycling, or swimming. After you're in shape, jogging, tennis, handball, soccer, or basketball are all acceptable forms of activity. But don't start off with high intensity exercises before your ligaments and bones have had a number of months of more gentle exercise progression. Minor injuries are common in the first months of a program. Sports such as football and baseball are not particularly good exercise and they aren't often practical for lifelong programs anyway.

Start off slowly. If you do not have a major medical problem, there is little point in a complete physical examination before exercising. After all, you're just going to be doing what the body was designed to do. If you have questions, mention to your doctor that you are in the process of starting a gradual exercise progression. Plan on at least five days a week, and at least 12 to 15 minutes of steady exercise each day. Your goal, which may take a year or more to achieve, is to have a morning resting pulse rate of less than 60 beats per minute. If you achieve this, you have good health, good cardiac reserve, and almost certainly have strengthened your musculoskeletal system to resist the aging process.

Common sense is the essential element. You can continue to increase your activity to any desired level including marathon running, mountain climbing, or other dramatic examples of intensive physical activity. But the benefits of exercise do *not* require heroic exercise programs. Every bit helps; the essential element is that a program be enjoyable and regular for life. It may take some time before you feel comfortable and easy about exercise, for old habits are hard to break. The euphoria that many exercisers report may not be experienced until the second or third year of a program. But you will have more zip in the evenings after only a few weeks or months. Health is its own reward.

CONTROL YOUR WEIGHT

Being overweight has many bad effects that we tend to forget. First, the extra weight places unnecessary stress on our weight-bearing joints. Second, the tendons and ligaments become separated by layers of fat and the leverage designed into your muscles and ligaments can't be smoothly applied. This results in more effort for a given task and creates tension on the ligament attachments from a direction for which they were not designed. So, episodes of bursitis and tendinitis are likely to result. Third, fat people are less active, although they often hate to admit it. Fourth, certain arthritis syndromes are much more common in the overweight. Low back pain is considerably more common in people who are obese, and some low-back-pain problems result from herniation of fat globules through back tissues. Some doctors feel that people with high triglycerides and high cholesterol develop certain kinds of arthritis. Surgery for obesity which bypasses the intestine can cause an arthritis. Fifth, fat-related diseases limit activity. These include diabetes, hernias, hemorrhoids, gallbladder problems, and even arteriosclerosis.

Weight control also requires lifetime discipline. You first need to establish your desired weight, usually the weight you held at about age 20. Basically, you need to eat less. The number of calories you take in must correspond with the calories you burn. You need to set intermediate goals for weight loss and you should integrate your exercise program with your weight-control program. Keep a graph of your progress toward your goals and achieve the goals on time. When you reach that bottom line, buy yourself new clothes and continue the graph, keeping your weight within five pounds of where you want to be. Expect some musculoskeletal pains during the weight-reduction phase and during the first few months at your ideal weight. These result from the tightening of the ligaments to the new dimensions of your body. They will go away and you will feel better. Don't let your weight go up and down like a yo-yo. Establish your desired weight and control it at that level.

Are you fat? Look in the mirror. Don't be overly concerned about meeting current norms for the ideal or "fashionable" weight. If you pinch the flesh around your middle and there is more than an inch between your thumb and forefinger, you are fat. And when you look in the mirror without any clothes on, it is hard to avoid the proper conclusion. Fight the tendency to rationalize ("I don't eat a thing"; "I have big bones"). You know better than that. The first step in controlling your weight is to confront the problem honestly. No particular diet is needed—just less of what you're having now. Cut out those elements in your present diet that are not particularly good for your body. Most of the "white" foods, such as breads and cakes and potatoes, can easily be dispensed with. Your goal is to maintain a balanced diet with foods from each of the major groups.

A caution against fad diets: The statistics on long-term weight reduction from any of the current or past fads are discouraging. Basically, the individual depends on the fad rather than on making the more difficult long-term commitment to weight control. Almost any diet, maintained enthusiastically, will take some weight off. The liquid-protein diet appears dangerous; other diets, although generally safe, are not a permanent answer. If you use them, you must also make the long-term, permanent commitment to weight control.

PROTECT YOUR JOINTS

The message of joint protection is to listen to the pain messages your body sends, and to do activities in the right way. Joints, ligaments, and bones can be damaged by misuse of a joint that is already inflamed or injured. Think of joint problems as being somewhat like a sprained ankle. The sprained ankle starts with an injury. There is pain and swelling and it may hurt to walk. Your body is attempting to repair the sprained ligament; the repair takes place most rapidly if you are easy on the joint during the repair period. If you are too active, you will sprain it again, and if you keep on spraining it, you can have a long-term problem. On the other hand, you can't let a sprained ankle destroy your life, so you need to continue some activity. So, you listen to the pain message. If it hurts a lot, don't do it. If it is reasonably comfortable, go ahead. This is simply common sense—and that is the essence of joint protection.

Warm up your muscles and joints before activity. Stretch your body and your joints through all their motions. Slowly increase your activities, as would an athlete in training. Don't forget your common sense.

Some injuries, such as a torn meniscus in the knee, a broken hip, or a broken finger, can accelerate later development of arthritis. So, avoiding activities likely to result in injury is another way of preventing arthritis. Football, baseball, and other activities that can result in injury do pose a hazard to the joints. Minor tendonitis, March fractures, and sprains may result from running or even walking; these do not lead to chronic arthritis.

In your exercise program, you are almost certain to develop some minor musculoskeletal problems. This *doesn't* mean that the exercise is not good. It does mean that you must use some restraint while exercising the injured part during its healing period.

Avoiding injury, listening to pain, wearing good shoes, maintaining good posture, and sleeping in a good bed are all methods of protecting the joints and preventing arthritis. In Part III we discuss specific techniques for protecting individual joints and for solving common problems.

PART

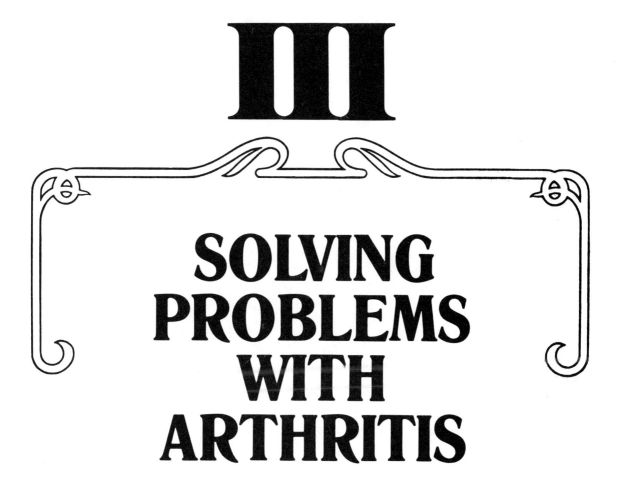

SOLVING PROBLEMS WITH ARTHRITIS

10

General Problems

1

Fatigue (Tiredness)

Most patients who have arthritis will experience some degree of fatigue. But most problems with fatigue are not physical weakness; they are related to depression, unhappiness, worry, or boredom. True weakness, as with inability to move an arm or a leg, is a physical problem involving the nerves, brain, or muscle and needs immediate medical attention. Fatigue is far more common.

Another common cause for fatigue is overuse of one drug or another. For example, caffeine, leading to poor sleep habits, can cause daytime fatigue. Or, tranquilizers can make you feel tired or drowsy. Once the normal sleep cycle has been disturbed, there is a tendency to grab an afternoon nap. Then, the following night's sleep is not good, because the afternoon nap decreased the need for sleep at night. A vicious cycle has been set in motion.

You may be assuming from this discussion that most fatigue is not serious. Usually, that's correct. Even when arthritis is associated, most fatigue results from misunderstanding your body. Reestablishing a pattern of healthy activity, more moderate drug use, and good nocturnal sleep will do wonders.

But, if your arthritis is an inflammatory one, such as rheumatoid arthritis or lupus, the disease may be causing the fatigue. This is a serious kind of fatigue and the measures above will not help much. In such cases the sed rate is elevated and there may be a low-grade fever. A hematocrit test may show the anemia of chronic disease. There may be some weight loss. Treatment of this kind of fatigue is based on treating the disease causing the fatigue; it may take some time to treat it correctly.

When you mention fatigue, most people don't even think of the problems listed above; they think of a problem with the thyroid, or of hypoglycemia, or of anemia. These are so unusual as causes of fatigue that you can almost forget about them. But if your fatigue persists more than six weeks despite home treatment, your doctor might want to check out these and other possibilities or may be able to reassure you that these problems are not present.

Fatigue is *not* old age. In fact, as you get older, you need less sleep and tend to be more alert, particularly early in the day. So, pay attention to this symptom.

Home Treatment

Listen to the fatigue message from your body. Heed it, but don't give in to it. Rest if you are tired, but alternate such periods with times of activity. Fatigue, because it can lead to physical deconditioning, can become its own cause.

Decrease all possible drugs including caffeine, nicotine, alcohol, tranquilizers, and probably TV! Pep pills can cause fatigue, as can Valium and codeine. Suspect everything.

Increase new activities. Friends, hobbies, travel, vacations, and even shopping tend to break the fatigue cycle. Increase your activity level by addition of smooth, graded, and easy exercises. Exercise helps you become involved in new and different things, as well as giving physical help by increasing your stamina.

Expect improvement to be slow and to be discouraged at times. Persevere.

What to Expect at the Doctor's Office

The topics noted above will be explored in depth at the doctor's office, with particular attention to the drugs being taken and associated psychological events. The nerves and muscles will be the focus of the physical examination. Blood tests, including thyroid tests, hematocrit, sed rate, and others, may be ordered. Probably no abnormality will be found. If your doctor doesn't think that tests are necessary, don't insist.

Treatment will be essentially as above. The doctor will treat the fatigue by treating the disease underlying. Do not expect pep pills, tonics, vitamins, or other magic. And be patient.

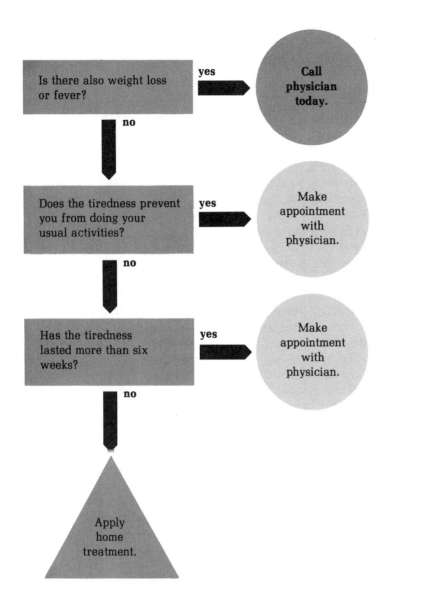

Is there also weight loss or fever?

yes → **Call physician today.**

no ↓

Does the tiredness prevent you from doing your usual activities?

yes → Make appointment with physician.

no ↓

Has the tiredness lasted more than six weeks?

yes → Make appointment with physician.

no ↓

Apply home treatment.

1
Fatigue (Tiredness)

2

Stiffness in the Morning

Morning stiffness is the hallmark of inflammatory rheumatic diseases. With a sprained ankle, with rheumatoid arthritis, with ankylosing spondylitis, or with other kinds of inflammation, you may notice that the sore area is stiff in the morning but loosens up as the day goes on. This phenomenon is most pronounced in rheumatoid arthritis and can be one of the patient's greatest aggravations.

No one really understands the reason for morning stiffness. Presumably, while the body is inactive, fluid leaks out from the small blood vessels and the tissues become waterlogged. Then, if you try to move the part, the swollen tissues feel stiff until the motion pumps the fluid out through the lymph channels and the veins. If you sit or lie down during the day, the stiffness will return. This phenomenon is called *gelling* or the *gel phenomenon* after the behavior of gelatin, which remains liquid if kept moving and warm but solidifies if it sits for long. The phenomenon appears to be normal, but in the patient with inflammatory arthritis it can be very vexing indeed.

Don't let morning stiffness keep you in bed. If your stiffness is that severe, call the doctor and discuss the problem today.

Home Treatment

With a local condition, such as a sprained ankle or a tennis elbow, don't worry about the stiffness. Think of it as a normal part of the process of bringing healing materials to the injured area. Loosen up carefully before activity and keep in mind that the healing is not yet complete. You should continue to protect the injured part.

With an inflammatory synovitis like rheumatoid arthritis (RA) the stiffness is apt to persist and you are going to have to come to grips with the problem. Use all of the tricks you can to reduce the inflammation and the stiffness.

Be sure that you take your prescribed medication according to schedule. The morning stiffness is a sign of the severity of the arthritis and the best way to reduce stiffness is to treat the arthritis. Your stiffness may be a signal that you have been sloppy in taking prescribed medication. Or, you may need more medication or a different drug. In particular, don't forget the last dose in the evening.

Ask your doctor about changing your medication schedule. Perhaps you can take a drug later in the evening or in the middle of the night, so that there is medication in your blood in the morning when you are most stiff. Indomethacin can be quite useful when added to other medication as a nighttime dose. If you are taking aspirin, some patients find that taking a coated aspirin (Ecotrin, Enseals) immediately before retiring helps reduce the morning stiffness. These coated aspirin are absorbed more slowly and the aspirin level lasts a bit longer. Avoid painkillers; they don't help morning stiffness.

Stretch gloves, of spandex or similar elastic material, may help morning stiffness if worn overnight. Give them a try; the idea is to prevent the tissues from becoming waterlogged. Try a warm bath or shower upon arising. Work at gentle exercises. You will have a certain amount of stiffness each day and you might as well get it worked out as soon as possible. Some people find that they are helped by using an electric blanket.

What to Expect at the Doctor's Office

The doctor's attention will be directed at control of the inflammation that is causing the stiffness. There may well be an increase in your prescribed medication or a change to a different set of treatments. For example, gold and penicillamine are two agents that are often helpful. Formal physical therapy is not likely to help, since the stiffness will have worked out by the time you reach the therapist. In inflammatory synovitis, increased morning stiffness is a signal for increased attention on the part of the doctor.

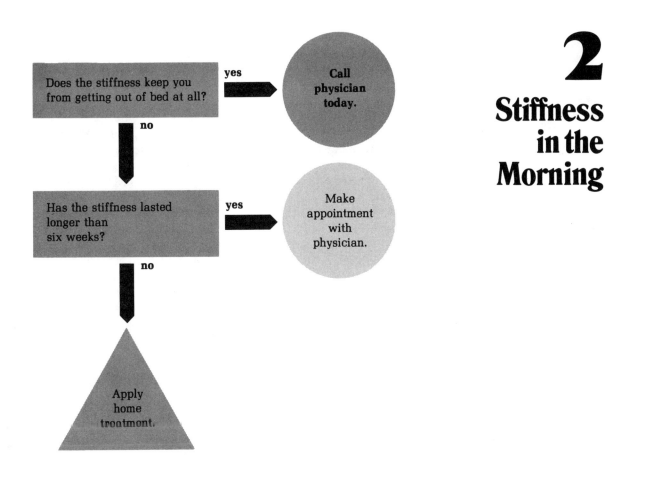

Does the stiffness keep you from getting out of bed at all?

yes → Call physician today.

no ↓

Has the stiffness lasted longer than six weeks?

yes → Make appointment with physician.

no ↓

Apply home treatment.

3

Weight Loss

Fortunately, weight loss is not very common with arthritis, but it is important when it occurs. A decline in weight that is not intentional and that results in falling below your ideal or normal weight is a signal that your body is not in equilibrium, that something substantial is wrong. Most people associate unwanted weight loss with cancer and may delay checking it out because they fear what might be found. This is not good thinking. Usually, weight loss is a problem that can be helped; this is particularly true of weight loss associated with arthritis.

For example, weight loss may be a clue to a depression. If you are a teenage girl or young woman, it may be *anorexia nervosa*, a psychiatric dysfunction that needs attention. It might be cancer, although usually not, but if it is, early treatment is especially important. An overactive thyroid can cause loss of weight, as can an infection, serious but easily treated, like tuberculosis. With a connective tissue disease, the arthritis condition can be causing the weight loss. Rheumatoid arthritis, polymyalgia rheumatica, lupus, polyarteritis, scleroderma, and polymyositis can all cause weight loss.

At any rate, weight loss is cause to see the doctor. An alarm bell has just rung. Check it out. It's hard to face the possibility of a major medical problem, but don't put it off.

Often a quite minor problem will be found. For example, difficulty in swallowing with scleroderma can result in weight loss and usually can be well treated. Or, a drug may be upsetting the stomach and some antacids and a change in medication will fix you up. Again, check it out.

Home Treatment

Not much of that here. Take care of yourself by going over this problem with your physician.

While getting checked out, there are a few things that you can do. Ask the doctor about stopping any medications that might be causing nausea, stomach pain, or loss of appetite. Codeine, Valium, aspirin, gold injections, penicillamine, and other drugs have these effects. If a drug has caused ulcers in the mouth, the doctor will surely want to stop it. If there is ulcer-like pain, antacids may be recommended. If you have the feeling of food sticking behind the breastbone, antacids again may be used to decrease the irritation to your esophagus. And don't forget to cut down on alcohol and coffee; these are two more drugs that are often overlooked.

What to Expect at the Doctor's Office

If depression is suspected, management will be that discussed later in problem 5. If the cause is not clear, a careful evaluation will be forthcoming. Often this means a number of tests and may even mean hospitalization. If the weight loss could be related to arthritis, tests such as rheumatoid factor (latex) or serum hepatitis antigen tests may be done. The thyroid may be checked. Chest X-ray, radiographs of the intestines, sigmoidoscopic examination (examination of the colon), and rectal examination may be needed. If you also have diarrhea, another set of tests are used to look for poor absorption of food. So, expect some attention when you go to the doctor with this complaint.

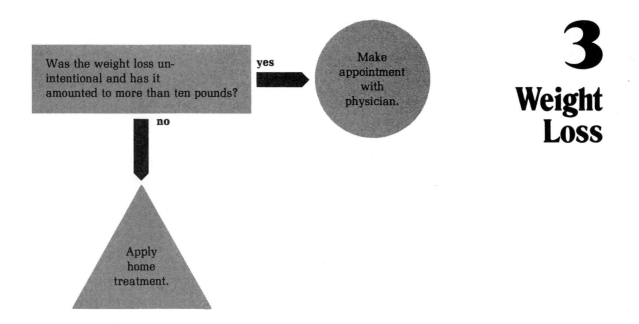

Was the weight loss un-intentional and has it amounted to more than ten pounds?

yes

Make appointment with physician.

no

Apply home treatment.

3
Weight Loss

4
Fever

Fever is not a disease. Rather, it is a symptom. It can mean anything or nothing, depending on its cause. In arthritis, fever can be a complicating infection in a joint or elsewhere or can be part of the disease, as in lupus, juvenile rheumatoid arthritis, or, more rarely, adult rheumatoid arthritis. Of course, people with arthritis get fever for all the same reasons that anybody else does, and most fever with arthritis should not be treated any differently than if the person did not have arthritis. With fever, management is based on the condition that is causing the fever, not the fever itself.

Here are some points to keep in mind. Watch out for fever from a bacterial infection. This kind of fever requires the most urgent attention, because antibiotics are necessary to treat the cause. Bacterial infections tend to be localized, and you usually can tell where the fever is coming from. It may be a sore throat, an earache, a boil, or a sore and swollen joint. Because of the way in which bacteria grow and divide, they are usually found in a single location, surrounded by pus cells—the body's response to the infection. With bacterial infections you may have a shaking chill. See the doctor if you suspect a bacterial infection. In contrast, viral infections tend to be less distinct; you may ache all over. These are less urgent, but any fever that persists for a long time should be checked out.

Arthritis-related fevers are few. Drug fever is the most common of these and you should always start by suspecting your medication. Rheumatoid arthritis occasionally causes low-grade fever, while lupus may show a more dramatic intermittent fever. Children with arthritis frequently have very high fevers indeed. Infectious arthritis, such as gonococcal arthritis, can cause fever. You can also get an infection in a joint already damaged by RA (or any other arthritis). Such infections are not common and often are discovered by an alert patient who notices that a single joint is acting up badly while other joints are doing well.

Duration separates out the serious fevers, so pay attention to how long your fever lasts, as noted on the decision chart.

Home Treatment

We have discussed fever and its treatment in detail in *Take Care of Yourself* and in *Taking Care of Your Child* (Addison-Wesley, 1977, 1978) and you may want to refer to those books for more complete treatment of this subject. Here, with the assumption of an underlying arthritis, the same general principles hold. You will usually be under the care of a doctor for your arthritis and you may want to give your doctor a call to check out your plan. If a drug might be causing the problem, ask about stopping the drug. For flu, minor fevers from viral illnesses, and other minor problems, you can take aspirin or acetaminophen in a dosage of ten grains (600 mg) every four hours. For children, the appropriate dose is one grain (60 mg) every four hours for each year of age up to age ten, then the adult dose. Of course, if you are already taking aspirin for your arthritis, a call to the doctor is in order. Keep the room cool. Wear light clothing. Children may require tepid baths to cool them down. Regular use of these measures is better and more comfortable than allowing the fever to go up and down like a yo-yo. If the fever might be related to the arthritis, you will want to see your doctor.

What to Expect at the Doctor's Office

Examination and culture of any suspicious area for bacteria can be expected. A joint may be "tapped" and cultured. X-rays may be taken if a suspected infection is located near bone. Antibiotics may be prescribed if a bacterial infection is known or strongly suspected. Antibiotics do not help viral infections and should not be given for uncomplicated colds or flu.

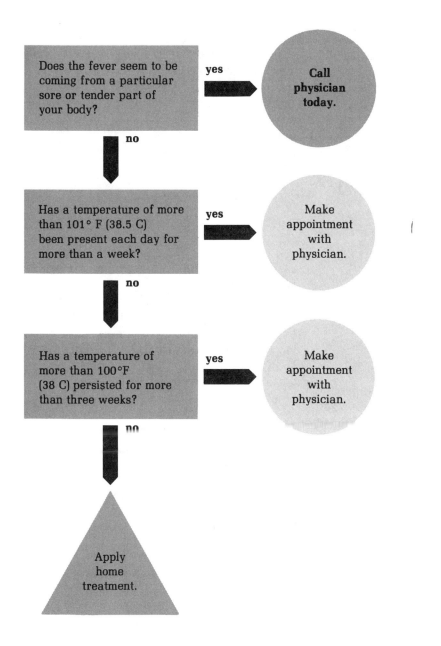

Does the fever seem to be coming from a particular sore or tender part of your body?

yes → Call physician today.

no ↓

Has a temperature of more than 101° F (38.5 C) been present each day for more than a week?

yes → Make appointment with physician.

no ↓

Has a temperature of more than 100°F (38 C) persisted for more than three weeks?

yes → Make appointment with physician.

no ↓

Apply home treatment.

4
Fever

5

Depression

Arthritis and depression are linked in the minds of many people. Perhaps this is because many of us associate arthritis with long-term pain, encroaching old age, or inevitability and hopelessness. Probably, the general perception that "little can be done" for arthritis contributes to these feelings of futility.

In fact, most kinds of arthritis compare very favorably with other human ills. Consider loss of eyesight, loss of a limb, a stroke, diabetes, anginal heart pains, heart failure, or emphysema. Most patients with arthritis do not have as major a medical problem as patients with one of these illnesses. Further, much more can be done for the arthritis. So, the hopelessness is mostly in our minds and the reality is far better than our common perceptions.

All patients with arthritis can lead satisfying lives. Arthritis should not cause a prolonged reactive depression. A few weeks or months of adjustment are to be expected with severe arthritis, but things should and will get better.

With depression, there is hopelessness. Unhappy thoughts flood the brain and you can't seem to shake them. You have trouble concentrating on anything for very long. You go to sleep all right but wake up early. Then you can't get back to sleep. Your speech and movements may be slow; your energy level is low. Your appetite is poor and you may lose weight. You may be constipated. You may have aches and increased stiffness. All of these problems will get better as the depression improves.

Most depression in arthritis is *reactive* (usually overreactive) depression—that is, the illness is precipitating the unhappiness. Or the depression may be due to drugs that have been given to treat the arthritis. From a psychiatric standpoint, these are not the worst kinds of depression; you can often work your own way out of them given a little time. There are some clear signals to seek professional help, however, and these are listed on the decision chart.

When unhappy, you may think briefly of suicide; this is almost normal. But if your reflections on suicide are serious or recurrent, or if you have actually considered the means by which you might commit suicide, it is essential that you seek help. Weight loss or unhappiness that shows no signs of improving after six weeks or more are also indications that you should see your physician.

Home Treatment

Check the drugs you are taking. The easiest way to cure a depression is to discover and stop the drug that is causing it. In particular, worry about the "downers" frequently used as tranquilizers. These can cause depression. Valium, Librium, and similar drugs have little, perhaps no, place in the treatment of arthritis. Codeine and other painkillers can also cause depression or aggravate it. Antihistamines can do the same. Even sleeping medications, because of the unnatural type of sleep they induce, can contribute to depression. Some arthritis medications, notably prednisone and indomethacin, can cause depressive reactions. If you suspect any of these, give the doctor a call or make a visit.

Increase activity and exercise. Friends, vacations, and new activities may need to be forced, but will help lift the depression. Change your pace. Start new hobbies. Do some things you've always wanted to do but kept putting off.

Project and anticipate future events. Find things to look forward to. Make long-range plans. Set intermediate goals. Work at living. Plan an exciting future event and begin saving and planning for it.

Know your limits. Get help when the signals are there. Most depressions ease and disappear if you work at life; a few don't and need some special care.

What to Expect at the Doctor's Office

A review of your medications and some changes, as well as discussion of the general factors mentioned above, can be expected.

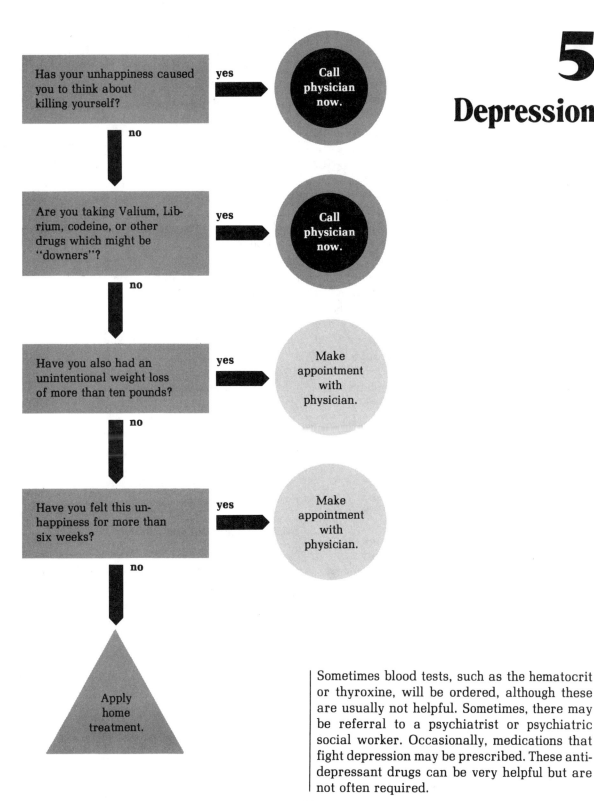

5

Depression

Has your unhappiness caused you to think about killing yourself?

yes → Call physician now.

no

Are you taking Valium, Librium, codeine, or other drugs which might be "downers"?

yes → Call physician now.

no

Have you also had an unintentional weight loss of more than ten pounds?

yes → Make appointment with physician.

no

Have you felt this unhappiness for more than six weeks?

yes → Make appointment with physician.

no

Apply home treatment.

Sometimes blood tests, such as the hematocrit or thyroxine, will be ordered, although these are usually not helpful. Sometimes, there may be referral to a psychiatrist or psychiatric social worker. Occasionally, medications that fight depression may be prescribed. These antidepressant drugs can be very helpful but are not often required.

6

Overweight (Obesity)

Throughout this book, you've no doubt repeatedly noticed the importance of weight control for your arthritis. Weight control is a difficult problem with no easy solutions. But it can be achieved. The principles of weight control are well established and, although you may not particularly enjoy it, you can successfully lose weight and keep it off.

First, check your diagnosis. Are you fat? Look at yourself naked in the mirror and be honest. Fat shows, and the mirror is more accurate than the tables of "normal" weights and heights. Your answer may be that you are not fat. Great! Just watch your weight from time to time; don't talk or worry about a problem that you don't have. Weight reduction and weight maintenance are life-and-death subjects; you can't afford to be dishonest with yourself or play social games with your friends about body weight.

Home Treatment

There are two steps to your program: weight reduction and weight maintenance. You must continue the maintenance program for the rest of your life—that's the hard part. So much for "fast" diets; weight control goes on forever. Fortunately, weight maintenance is possible with over 95 percent of the calories that you would eat if you were fat and gaining. So, while you need some privation, you do not need to starve yourself.

For weight reduction, almost any popular diet that is reasonably safe is all right. (Avoid liquid-protein diets; these are not safe.) Or, you can just eat less. Don't eat anything between dinner and breakfast, have less high-calorie alcohol, decrease white carbohydrates (sugar, breads, cakes, potatoes), stop desserts and snacks, and exercise more. Remember that a lot of weight-control programs are undermined by impulse buying in the supermarket—what you don't bring home you can't eat.

Usually, a weight loss of about a pound a week is a good pace, even if you have forty or fifty pounds to lose. You are in this for the long haul. Set early, intermediate, and long-term goals. Write them down. Tell others about them. Commit yourself! Get a good scale and plot your weight every week on a chart. Same day, same time, same scale, same clothing. Note progress toward your goal. Keep at it. Expect your rate of weight loss to slow down after a few days—the first pounds are mostly water and give you a false sense of progress anyway. Remember, total starvation results in a weight loss of only about one pound a day, so any change greater than this simply represents a fluid shift that can reverse itself just as quickly. Over the long term, your graph will show your progress. Weight loss groups, such as Weight Watchers, can be a big help.

What to Expect at the Doctor's Office

Your doctor should give you the same advice that you have just read. Motivation and perseverance—not any magic treatments—are the keys to weight loss and maintenance. Pills are not useful for weight loss and can be hazardous. This is a home-treatment problem. Don't keep chasing the rainbow; get to work.

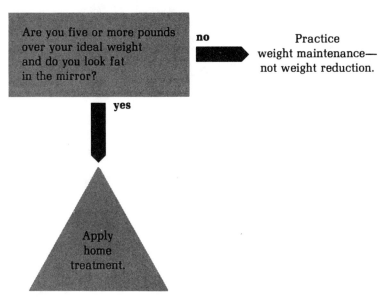

Are you five or more pounds over your ideal weight and do you look fat in the mirror?

no → Practice weight maintenance— not weight reduction.

yes ↓

Apply home treatment.

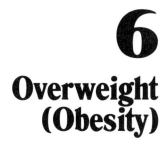

6
Overweight (Obesity)

11

Problems with Pain

7
Pain in the Ball of the Foot

The sole of your shoe wears at the "ball" of your foot, and your shoe may get a hole in it at that point. It wasn't true for our four-footed ancestors, but this is the point of greatest stress when we walk. We even make it worse by footwear designed for fashion rather than function. And, unfortunately, this area is where the metatarsal bones join the toe bones; there are five important joints in each foot in this region. At these "MTP" or metatarsal-phalangeal joints, occurs a great proportion of the arthritis that affects the foot.

The consequences of arthritis in the forefoot (*metatarsalgia*) are major and adverse. With every step, we place weight on this area, and it is difficult indeed to walk without using the forefoot. Even a small problem can make walking difficult, and other muscles, tendons, ligaments, and bones begin to lose strength. Serious attention by you is required, because careful work at home can pay major dividends. Even though your arthritis is a systemic synovitis, you will find that attention to local factors can make all the difference.

Very rarely, you may have one of the indications on the decision chart to call your doctor. These questions are to make sure that you don't have gout, an infection, an unstable fracture, or nerve damage. Usually you won't, and this is then a home-treatment problem.

Home Treatment

The solution is usually quite simple. The principle is to move the weight bearing away from the painful part, so that the inflammation can subside. The *metatarsal bar*, a strip of sole leather that the shoemaker will sew or glue on about an inch behind the area where you are wearing the sole, is the key device to shift your weight. An insert in the shoe takes up room in the shoe, and most toes with arthritis need more room rather than less; but these help a few people and have the advantage that they can be transferred from shoe to shoe. The metatarsal bar goes on the outside. When you check your area of greatest pain against the area of greatest wear on the shoe, you will find that they are the same. Press on your foot about an inch behind the sore place and you will note how much better it feels and the way that the toes line up straighter. The metatarsal bar will also help your arch. It is an inexpensive device and any good shoemaker knows how to fit one. Fix several pairs of shoes.

Shoes are critical to problems of foot pain. Don't wear shoes with pointed toes. Avoid high heels—they throw additional weight on the forefoot. Look for a wide toe box. You can tell a lot in the store by walking around before buying; don't go home with a purchase that isn't comfortable, no matter what the salesperson says. Ask particularly to try the "Duckbill" made by the Joyce company or the "Roundabout" by Dr. Scholl. These shoes have a wide toe box and are comfortable for most; they are readily available and their cost is much less than that of specially made shoes. Try the athletic shoe department for casual shoes. The newer shoes designed for long-distance running on pavement are excellent for arthritis and should be more widely used; they are comfortable and relatively inexpensive. Look for shoes with a good heel wedge support, a nylon upper that will spread in the toe box, and laces that run through guides rather than eyelets, so that they adjust smoothly. Brooks Vantage and New Balance 320 are two good brands, but there are others as well.

If your problem with pain in the forefoot occurs at night, you will need something to raise the covers off the foot. A pillow under the covers at the bottom of the bed is the easiest solution; a side-lying L-shaped piece of wood may be better for tall folks.

What to Expect at the Doctor's Office

The doctor will examine your foot and ankle, and sometimes take an X-ray. Advice will be much the same as that given above. Injection is

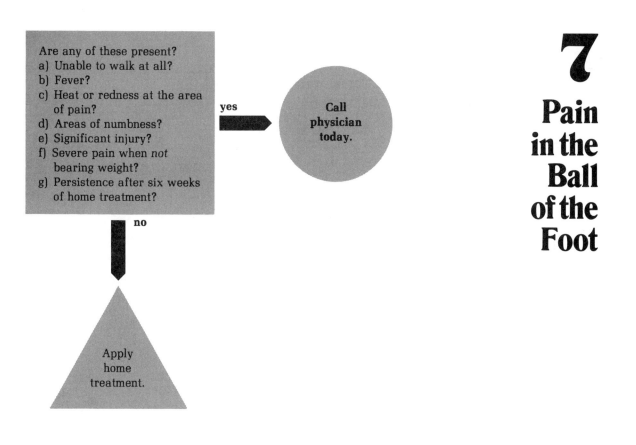

Are any of these present?
a) Unable to walk at all?
b) Fever?
c) Heat or redness at the area of pain?
d) Areas of numbness?
e) Significant injury?
f) Severe pain when *not* bearing weight?
g) Persistence after six weeks of home treatment?

yes → Call physician today.

no

Apply home treatment.

7

Pain in the Ball of the Foot

occasionally of some use. Fancy shoes may be ordered, but if you have followed the instructions under "Home Treatment," you are likely to be disappointed when the $300 shoes aren't as comfortable as those selected in a shoestore. If problems are persistent, surgery is sometimes required and is often well worthwhile.

Bunionectomy, metatarsal head resection, and resection of a Morton's neuroma (tumor) are three frequently useful procedures. The operation for putting plastic joints in the forefoot is not yet perfected. Finally, your doctor may increase anti-inflammatory medications to improve the underlying arthritis.

8

Pain in the Heel

Heel pain can occur at one of two places; the bottom of the heel or the back of the heel. The heel bone, the calcaneus, is the largest bone of the foot and bears our full weight during part of each stride. The painful heel, in almost all instances, is caused by excessive strain on one of the two major ligaments, and the pain occurs where these ligaments attach. The achilles tendon attaches at the back of the heel. This is the strongest tendon in the body and connects the muscles on the back of the calf to the heel. The force of contraction of the muscles enables us to stand on tiptoe and gives an extra thrust as we walk or run. Damage to this tendon attachment is called Achilles tendinitis. Frequently there will also be tears in the tendon itself or in the lower part of the muscle.

The heel-spur syndrome affects the bottom of the heel. This is where the ligaments that make up the arch of the foot attach to the heel bone. These ligaments function like a bowstring to arch the foot, so you can see that they are under pressure every time we stand or step. If the problem persists, calcium may develop in the inflamed area where the ligaments attach. The presence of the calcium spur may or may not cause additional pain; often the spur itself is only the visible part of a painful process. Many people have pain without visible spurs, while others have spurs but no pain.

Heel pain of both back and bottom type can occur in Reiter's syndrome or ankylosing spondylitis. Here the process is the same except that no injury is required and rest is not as effective a treatment. Even more rarely, gout or infection will be present. Usually, heel pain is the simple result of a forgotten injury.

Home Treatment

Rest, avoidance of further injury, and gradual resumption of activity as the pain subsides are indicated. Activities not requiring weight bearing, like swimming, can be continued full tilt.

For Achilles tendinitis, rest the foot or feet. Use a shoe with a high heel wedge and a lot of padding, since this limits the stretch on the tendon. Warm up carefully for ten or fifteen minutes before activities that might cause reinjury and avoid sudden starts, particularly on cold days. Tennis and running uphill are not good. Remember that tight muscles on the back of the leg put extra strain on this tendon, so warm up with toe-touching or hurdler-position exercises.

For the heel-spur syndrome, treatment is just the same, except that the activities to avoid are ones that cause pounding on the bottom of the heel. Heel padding will help, but support for the arch is even more important, since this takes tension off the ligaments whose job it is to hold the arch. Shoes should be selected according to the criteria discussed in problem 7, except that a large toe box is not essential. My favorite is the Brooks Vantage or a similar running shoe with a very thick heel and excellent arch. Don't worry about wearing a "silly-looking" shoe around—forget fashion and concentrate on getting well.

After six weeks of treatment, check with your doctor if you are still having trouble.

What to Expect at the Doctor's Office

Your doctor will examine the painful areas and give you advice like that above. If Reiter's syndrome or ankylosing spondylitis is present, major relief may be obtained from indomethacin or other nonsteroidal anti-inflammatory agents. These drugs should not be used for injuries as a rule, since they suppress the healing inflammatory response. Injection of steroids into the Achilles tendon area is quite dangerous and should be avoided; the entire tendon will sometimes rip apart after an injection has weakened it. Some doctors have found it helpful to scrape the heel spur off the underlying bone with a needle or a knife.

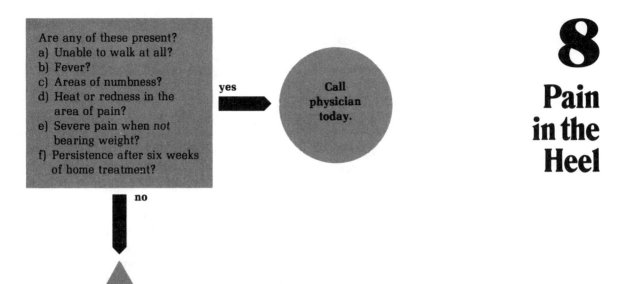

Are any of these present?
a) Unable to walk at all?
b) Fever?
c) Areas of numbness?
d) Heat or redness in the area of pain?
e) Severe pain when not bearing weight?
f) Persistence after six weeks of home treatment?

yes

Call physician today.

no

Apply home treatment.

8
Pain in the Heel

9

Pain in the Ankle

The ankle is a large joint, with lots of synovium to get inflamed. Since it is a weight-bearing joint, it is unavoidably stressed at each step. As a result, synovitis is usually not the direct cause of pain or instability of the ankle joint. Most frequently, the problem is in the ligaments near the joint. The sprained ankle is a simple example of this. With an ankle sprain, the ligament attaching the bump on the outer side of the ankle to the outer surface of the foot is injured at one or both ends. The ankle itself is all right. With rheumatoid arthritis, the synovitis may have injured the adjacent ligaments so that the joint slips, ligaments are strained, and pain and instability result. Walking on an unstable joint just increases the damage, but if you can stabilize the joint, walking is usually all right.

If you look down your leg when lying and when standing you can tell if the joint is stable. If it is unstable, the line of weight going down your leg will not be straight down the foot. Perhaps the foot will be slipped a half inch or an inch to the outside of where it should be. When you are not bearing weight, it will move back in line toward a more normal position. The unstable joint may actually slip sideways if you try to move the foot with your hands.

Rarely, infection or gout may be the cause of this problem; the questions on the decision chart are designed to minimize this possibility.

Home Treatment

Listen to the pain message: it is telling you to rest the part a bit more, to provide support for the unstable ankle, to back off on your exercise progression, or to use an aid to take weight off the ankle.

The unstable ankle should be supported for major weight-bearing activity. Instability is not just a swollen ankle; the ankle must be displaced sideways or be crooked. Support is most simply obtained by high-lacing boots, but sometimes these will be too uncomfortable and you will have to have specially made boots or an ankle brace. Professional help is required for adequate fitting of such devices and they can be quite expensive.

For the stable ankle, an elastic bandage and a shoe with a comfortable, thick heel pad will help; the jogging shoes described in problems 7 and 8 are good.

Crutches are often a big help for a flare-up, and even a cane can help you take weight off the sore ankle. Remember to have the crutches short enough so as not to injure the nerves in your armpits by leaning on the crutch; take the weight on your hands or arms.

If you have a synovitis, then make sure that you have been taking your medication exactly as prescribed. Sometimes a patient gets a little bored and lax with the pill-taking routine and, a few days later, experiences difficulty walking because of pain or swelling.

As soon as the pain begins to decrease, you can gently begin to exercise the joint again. Swimming is good, because you don't have to bear weight. Start easy and slow with your exercises. Sit on a chair, let the leg hang free, and wiggle the foot up and down and in and out. Later, walk carefully with an ankle bandage for support. Stretch the ankle by pulling the forefoot on a step and lowering the heel. As the ankle gains strength, you can walk on tiptoe and walk on your heels to stretch and strengthen the joint. Do the exercises several times a day; the ankle shouldn't be a lot worse after the exercise if you aren't overdoing. Keep at it but take your time.

What to Expect at the Doctor's Office

The doctor will examine the painful area and may take X-rays. The dose of anti-inflammatory

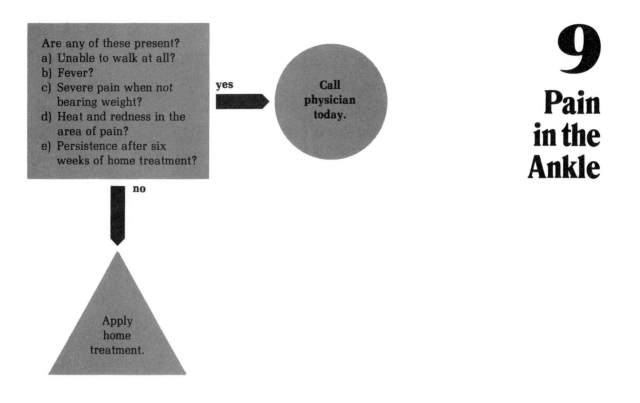

Are any of these present?
a) Unable to walk at all?
b) Fever?
c) Severe pain when *not* bearing weight?
d) Heat and redness in the area of pain?
e) Persistence after six weeks of home treatment?

yes → Call physician today.

no ↓

Apply home treatment.

9

Pain in the Ankle

drugs may be increased. Special shoes or braces may be prescribed. Surgery is occasionally necessary. Fusion (non-motion) of the ankle is the most generally useful procedure; a fixed, pain-free ankle is far preferable to an unstable and painful one. The artificial ankle joint is not yet satisfactory for most people, but progress is rapid in this area.

181

10
Pain in the Knee

The knee is a hinge. It is, of course, a large, weight-bearing joint. But it is a hinge, and its motion is much more strictly limited than that of most other joints. It will straighten to make the leg a stable support and it will bend (flex) to more than a right angle (120°). However, it will not move in any other direction. The limited motion of the knee gives it great strength, but it is not engineered to take side stresses, as football players discover repeatedly each year.

There are two cartilage compartments in each knee—one inner and one outer. If the cartilage wears unevenly, the leg can bow in or out. Or, if you are born with crooked legs, there can be strain that causes the cartilage to wear more rapidly.

The knee must be stable and it must be able to extend fully to a straight leg. If it lacks full extension, the muscles have to support the body at all times and strain is continuous; normally our knee "locks" in the straight position and allows us to rest (or a horse to sleep standing up). If the knee wobbles from side to side, there is too much stress on the side ligaments and the condition will gradually worsen.

If the knee is unstable and wobbles or if it cannot be straightened out, you need the doctor. Similarly, you need a physician if there is a possibility of gout or an infection; the knee is the joint most frequently bothered by these serious problems. Finally, if there is pain or swelling in the calf below the sore knee, you may have a blood clot, but more likely you have a *Baker cyst* and you need the doctor. These cysts start as fluid-filled sacs in an inflamed knee but enlarge through the tissues of the calf and may cause swelling quite a distance below the knee.

Home Treatment

Listen to the pain message and try not to do things that aggravate the pain either imme-diately or the next day. If there has been a recent injury, then an elastic bandage may help; otherwise, probably not. Use of a cane can help; the cane is best carried in the hand on the side of the painful knee by some, while others carry it on the opposite side.

Do *not* use a pillow under the knee at night or at any other time, as this can make the knee stiffen so that it cannot be straightened out.

Exercises should be started slowly and performed several times daily if possible. Swimming is good because there is no weight-bearing requirement. From the beginning pay close attention to flexing and straightening the leg. A friend can help, since it may be more comfortable to move the leg passively. But work at getting it straight and keeping it straight. Next, begin isometric exercises. Tense the muscles in your upper leg, front and back, at the same time, so that you are exerting force but your leg is not moving. Exert force for two seconds, then rest two seconds. Do ten repetitions three times a day. Then, begin gentle, active exercises. A bicycle in a low gear is a good place to start. Or, walk for short distances. *Avoid* deep knee bends; they place too much stress on the knee.

Knee problems can come from the feet, as in jogging or tennis. Proper shoes, as advised in problems 7 and 8, can help.

Make sure that you are taking your medication as directed, since your painful knee could be caused by too little medication.

What to Expect at the Doctor's Office

Examination of the knee, other joints, and possibly an X-ray of the knee. If a Baker cyst is suspected, or for diagnostic reasons, some fluid may be drawn from the knee through a needle and tested. This procedure is easy, not too uncomfortable, and quite safe. If you have an unstable knee after an injury, you may need surgery to repair the torn ligaments or remove the torn cartilage. If you have synovitis, a synovectomy (removal of the synovium) may be recommended. This can be useful, but it is an

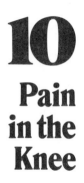

10
Pain in the Knee

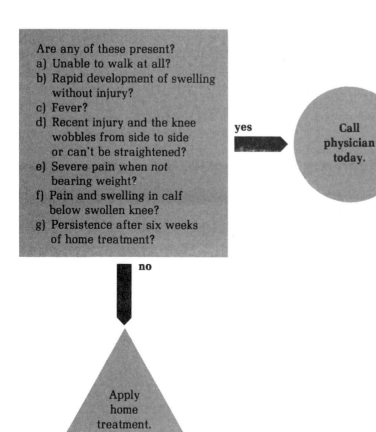

Are any of these present?
a) Unable to walk at all?
b) Rapid development of swelling without injury?
c) Fever?
d) Recent injury and the knee wobbles from side to side or can't be straightened?
e) Severe pain when *not* bearing weight?
f) Pain and swelling in calf below swollen knee?
g) Persistence after six weeks of home treatment?

yes → Call physician today.

no ↓

Apply home treatment.

operation you may want to get a second opinion about. For severe problems, total knee replacement may be recommended. This is a good operation and usually gives total pain relief. Other operations include removal of bits of bone or cartilage (joint mice), and removal of some bone (osteotomy) in order to straighten the leg.

11

Pain in the Hip

The hip is a "ball-and-socket" joint. The largest bone in the body, the femur, is in the thigh, and narrows to a neck that angles in to the pelvis and ends in a ball-shaped knob. This ball fits into a curved socket in the pelvic bone (acetabulum). This arrangement provides a joint that can move freely in all directions. The joint itself is located rather deeply under some big muscles so that it is protected from dislocating—that is, from coming out of the socket.

Two new problems arise because of this arrangement of the anatomy. The neck of the femur can break rather easily, and this is usually what happens when an older person "breaks a hip" after a slight fall. Also, the "ball" part of the joint must get its blood supply from below, and the small artery that supplies the "head" of the femur can get clogged, leading to death of the bone and a kind of arthritis called *aseptic necrosis*.

The hip joint can also get infected and, rarely, it will be the site for an attack of gout. The bursae that lie over the joint can be inflamed with a bursitis. True synovitis, as in rheumatoid arthritis, can injure the joint. And, it is not uncommon for attachment arthritis, such as ankylosing spondylitis, to cause stiffness or loss of motion at the hip.

A *flexion contracture* means that motion at the hip joint has been partly lost. The hip becomes partially fixed in a slightly bent position. When walking or standing, this causes the pelvis to tilt forward, so that when you stand straight, the back has to curve a little extra. This throws strain on the low back area.

For poorly understood reasons, pain in the hip is often felt down the leg, often at the knee or just above. This is called *referred pain*. Nonreferred hip pain may be felt in the groin or the upper, outer thigh. Pain that starts in the low back is often felt in the region of the hip.

Since the hip joint is so deeply located, it can often be troublesome to locate the exact source of pain in these regions.

Home Treatment

Listen for the pain message and try to avoid activities that are painful or aggravate pain. You will want to avoid pain medication as much as possible. Rest the joint from painful activities. Use a cane or crutches if necessary. The cane is usually best held in the hand opposite to the painful hip, since this allows greater relaxation in the large muscles around the hip joint. Move the cane and the affected side simultaneously, then the good side, then repeat.

As the pain begins to resolve, exercise should be gradually introduced. First, use gentle motion exercises to free the hip and prevent stiffness. Stand with your good hip by a table and lean on the table with your hand. Let the bad hip swing to and fro and front and back. Lie on your back with your body half off the bed and the bad hip hanging, and let the leg stretch backward toward the floor. See how far apart you can straddle your legs, and bend the upper body from side to side. Try to turn your feet apart like Charlie Chaplin, so that the rotation ligaments get stretched. Repeat these exercises gently three times a day.

Then, introduce more active exercises to strengthen the muscles around the hips. Lie on your back and raise your legs. Swimming stretches muscles and builds good muscle tone. Bicycle or walk. When walking, start with short strides and gradually lengthen them as you loosen up. Gradually increase your effort and distance, but not by more than 10 percent each day. A good firm bed will help, and the best sleeping position is on your back. Avoid pillows beneath the knees or under the low back.

Make sure you are taking anti-inflammatory medication as prescribed if you have a synovitis or an attachment arthritis.

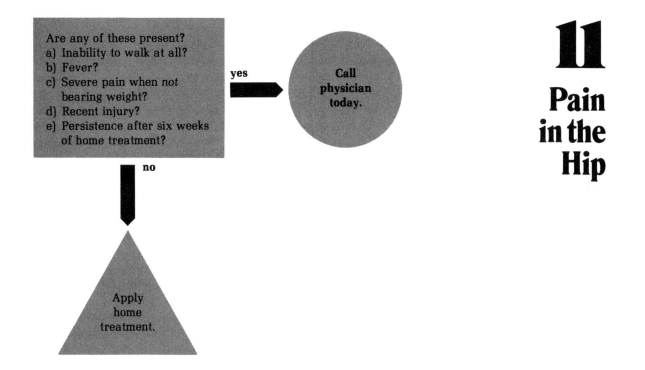

Are any of these present?
a) Inability to walk at all?
b) Fever?
c) Severe pain when *not* bearing weight?
d) Recent injury?
e) Persistence after six weeks of home treatment?

yes → Call physician today.

no

Apply home treatment.

11

Pain in the Hip

What to Expect at the Doctor's Office

Expect examination of the hip and motion of the hip, as well as your other joints and your back. X-rays may be taken. Anti-inflammatory medication may be increased. Injection is only rarely used or needed. One of several surgical procedures may be recommended if the pain is bad and persistent or if you are having real problems walking. Total hip replacement, a remarkable new operation, has largely superseded many older techniques. This is almost always successful in stopping pain and may help mobility a great deal. The artificial hip should last at least 10 or 15 years with current techniques. You get up and around quite quickly after surgery and the complications are rather rare. Other procedures include pinning of the hip, replacing either the ball or the socket, but not both, or removing a wedge of bone to straighten out the joint angle.

12

Pain in the Lower Back

Lower back pain—practically a universal problem—is discussed in Part I (on page 71). The crucial things to remember are that this problem is common (most people get it), painful (incredibly), medically minor (most of the time), and that the cause is nearly always an injury that requires times to heal completely. Medication cannot speed the healing process. If there is any sign of nerve damage, or if a fracture might have occurred, or if it just won't go away, see the doctor.

Home Treatment

Think again of a sprained ankle. The injury causes bruising and swelling for two or three days, then slow healing begins to become evident. Pain is better in less than a week, but six weeks is required for full healing. Reinjury is costly, since the healing process must start again from the beginning. Low back pain is the same.

Do not take all kinds of pain killers and muscle relaxants and then go on as if your back was all right; this practice has a high likelihood of reinjury. Either take the medication and rest flat in bed, or listen to the pain message and do only what you can do in reasonable comfort.

Don't apply heat to the area the first day; if anything, use cold packs to decrease pain and swelling. Heat may be cautiously applied after the first day, but it really won't help a lot. A firm mattress or a bed board is part of the standard advice; back problems vary, however, and if you are more comfortable at night and the following morning with a slightly softer mattress, use that. Aspirin or other mild pain relievers are probably all right, but they won't help too much. A small pillow or folded towel beneath the lower back may increase your comfort when sleeping flat. When you get up,

draw your knees up, then roll sideways and sit up. The position of lying on your side, knees up, is more comfortable than the back for many people and it is all right.

You doubtless have muscle spasms. Although painful, they are protecting your injured back. If you can last out the discomfort without muscle relaxants and without a lot of pain medication, your back may heal more strongly and you decrease the chance of reinjury.

Exercises shouldn't be started for a week or so, until things feel a lot better, and then they should be begun slowly. Exercise is designed to make recurrence less likely by toning the muscles and ligaments so that the spine has greater strength. Abdominal muscles assist spinal stability and are part of the exercise program. If you have some weight to lose, get started with the weight reduction right away.

Exercises should be repeated several times daily and gradually increased in number and in effort expended. Toe-touching, side-bending, and twisting exercises are not particularly good; for the back you are more interested in strength than suppleness. Here are two good exercises: (1) Lie on the back and tighten the stomach muscles so that the hollow of the back is forced against the floor. Tense and hold for two seconds, relax, and repeat three times. Gradually work up to ten repetitions. (2) Lie on your back, pillow under your head. Hug your knees to your chest with your hands, exhale so that your spine can curve as much as possible, hold for five seconds, relax, and repeat 3 times. Work up to ten repetitions.

Posture helps. Sit in a straight chair. Keep your shoulders back. Have a good mattress on your bed. (Water beds, surprisingly, usually work out very well.) Lift weight with your legs, not your back. Never lift from a bending forward position. Avoid sudden shifts and strains, particularly those that throw the upper body backwards. Tennis, for example, should not be rushed as your back recovers. You can safely walk, swim, or bicycle long before it would be safe to resume your tennis game.

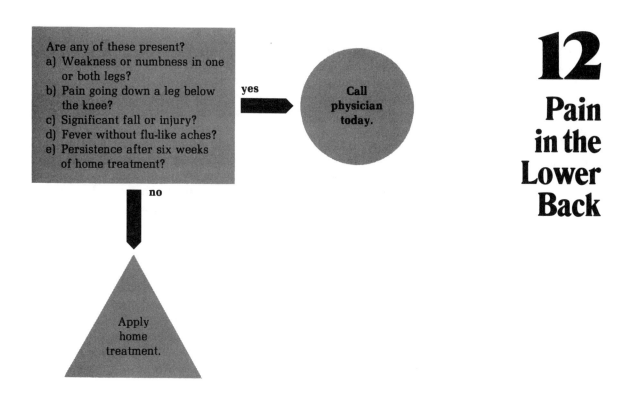

Are any of these present?
a) Weakness or numbness in one or both legs?
b) Pain going down a leg below the knee?
c) Significant fall or injury?
d) Fever without flu-like aches?
e) Persistence after six weeks of home treatment?

yes → Call physician today.

no ↓

Apply home treatment.

12
Pain in the Lower Back

What to Expect at the Doctor's Office

Unfortunately, don't expect too much. Unless there is nerve injury, the doctor doesn't have much to offer. Surgery is best reserved for patients with nerve-compression syndromes or for particularly severe and persistent difficulties. As most people know, failure of surgery to improve back problems is rather common.

The commonly used drug regimens of painkillers and muscle relaxants have never been shown to shorten the time of recovery or to help prevent recurrence; there is reason to suppose that under some circumstances these drugs can increase the chance of reinjury and can thereby delay healing. These drugs also affect your thinking processes and offer some hazard if you drive a car or operate heavy machinery. Uncomplicated low back strain is a problem for home treatment first.

If there is nerve injury traction or surgery can help and your delay in seeking medical care could have permanent consequences. So, keep looking for the danger signs of weakness, numbness, or pain going down the leg below the knee.

13

Pain in the Neck

Someone is a "pain in the neck" if they just keep on bothering you and won't go away. Neck pain is thus so memorable that it has reference in folk idiom. Most people have neck pain at some point and, occasionally, a person has quite serious problems.

The neck bones are a continuation of the spine. The top seven vertebrae are called cervical or neck vertebrae. The seventh one makes the prominent bump you can feel where your back joins your neck. The uppermost vertebra, the atlas, holds up the skull. The second vertebrae, the axis, has a vertical peg (odontoid), around which the head turns. The entire neck is more flexible than the back; it bears less weight but is less well protected by thick muscles. The disk spaces in the neck can get narrow, bony spurs can form, and nerves can get caught and compressed, just as in the low back. Spondylitis and other forms of attachment arthritis can affect the neck, and rheumatoid arthritis is particularly likely to affect the top two vertebrae, allowing the head to slip forward and backward on the neck. Injuries to the ligaments of the neck take some time to heal.

Usually, like the low back, a neck problem is minor and will be self-limited. It must depend on natural healing processes to resolve. Excessive neck movement tends to slow the healing and has the possibility of causing reinjury.

Home Treatment

Rest the neck and listen for what the pain message tells you not to do. You can take a bath towel, fold it lengthwise so that it is a four-inch wide strip, and wrap the neck with it, securing it comfortably with a safety pin or tape. Now you have a soft neck brace to wear at night, and this will clear up nearly half of all neck-pain problems. If things persist, use the soft collar during the day as well or buy a commercial soft collar to wear. You want some support from the collar, but more than that you want a little reminder not to turn your head too fast or too far.

Watching a tennis match is obviously not a good idea, because of the repeated head turning required. You probably engage in other activities just as damaging without realizing it. For example, wearing your glasses while reading may decrease the neck movements required, because you will be farther away from the book. Sit back farther from your work. Common sense says to watch out for things that aggravate the pain and to stop doing them.

Keep painkillers and muscle relaxants to a minimum or avoid them altogether. Aspirin or acetaminophen is all right but won't make you feel much better. Sleep on a good firm mattress. Don't sleep on your stomach, and if you sleep on your side, place a pillow so that your neck is in a neutral position, not propped up or hanging down. On your back, move the pillow beneath your neck as well as your head and keep the pillow a small one. Don't reach or look over your head to get objects; use a stool.

Exercises begin as the pain subsides, usually after five to seven days. Don't rush them—they are designed to help prevent the next recurrence. There are two types of exercise, the stretching exercises and the strength exercises, and you should do some of each. Start stretching exercises with gentle stretches and increase the stretch slowly day by day. Do them twice daily, each maneuver three times. There are three exercises: chin toward chest, ear toward shoulder, and look to the side. The last two should of course be done in each direction.

Strength exercises can begin at the same time and start with three repetitions twice daily. Slowly work up to ten repetitions. If you have been having recurrent neck problems, the exercises are a worthwhile lifetime habit. Here are three: (1) Shoulder shrug—raise both shoulders toward ears, hold for two seconds, relax, repeat. (2) Take a deep, deep breath, hold for five seconds, release, repeat. The neck muscles are "accessory muscles of respiration" and breathing exercises involve the neck. (3) While standing, grab one thumb with your other hand with both hands behind your back.

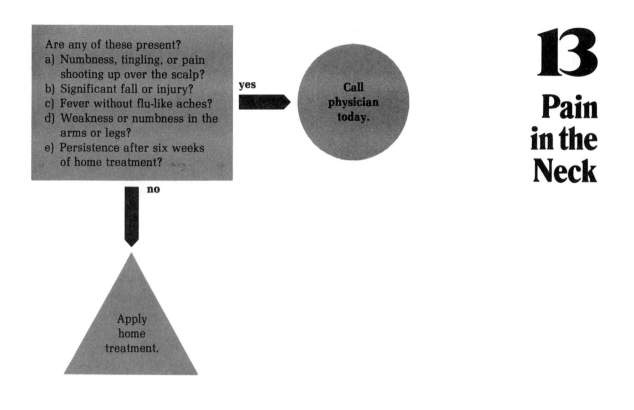

Are any of these present?
a) Numbness, tingling, or pain shooting up over the scalp?
b) Significant fall or injury?
c) Fever without flu-like aches?
d) Weakness or numbness in the arms or legs?
e) Persistence after six weeks of home treatment?

yes

Call physician today.

no

Apply home treatment.

13

Pain in the Neck

Flex your head way back. Press down with your hand. Take a deep breath, relax, repeat. This exercise can be done lying on your stomach as well, after you get good at it standing up.

A hot shower may increase comfort while exercising. Some authorities recommend doing the exercises in the shower.

What to Expect at the Doctor's Office

The uncomplicated neck-pain problem is a job for home treatment first. If there is pressure on a nerve, then hospitalization, traction, myelograms, and surgery may be needed, but if there is no nerve pressure, the doctor has relatively little additional advice to offer. Surgery in the neck is inconsistent in relieving the problem. If your long-term neck problem doesn't have any "objective" findings and X-rays don't reveal a physical problem, a visit to a psychiatrist may be recommended. Tension headaches are a simple emotional problem that can localize in the neck muscles. Similarly, other psychiatric syndromes sometimes underlie a pain in the neck that just won't go away.

14

Pain in the Shoulder

When the shoulder is affected by a problem, it has a tendency to become "frozen," regardless of the nature of the problem. The frozen shoulder is stiff, limited in motion, and can be permanent if not appropriately treated. Understanding the way the shoulder works will help you understand the many different injuries that result in the same general problem.

The shoulder is our largest non-weight-bearing joint and has a complicated set of motions. Actually, the motions come from a series of three different joints that, in combination, give us the ability to swing our arms every which way, together with reasonable strength and stability at the joint.

If you lift your arm straight up over your head, you can feel the three joints come into play one after the other by using your other hand to feel the movement of the bones. The first 90° of motion, from arm-at-the-side to arm-straight-out-to-the-side, come from the true shoulder joint. This joint is a shallow ball and socket held together by a tough fibrous capsule, lined with synovial cells and covered over with tendons and muscles. It connects the arm to the shoulder blade.

As you raise your arm higher, the shoulder blade begins to move, because of motion at a fibrous joint that joins the shoulder blade to the collarbone. This allows perhaps 75° more of motion. Finally, the entire collarbone begins to tilt up, moving at a fibrous joint connecting the collarbone to the breastbone. This intricate design permits more motion at the shoulder joint than at any other joint.

An injury of any kind tends to immobilize this complex apparatus, and the inflammation that is helping repair the damage can involve nearby tissues. As healing occurs, adhesions may stick surfaces together and motion can be permanently lost—hence, the frozen shoulder.

This stiffening process is much more common in the shoulder than in any other joint.

The causes can be many: athletic injury, calcific tendonitis, rheumatoid arthritis, aseptic necrosis, ankylosing spondylitis, and many other conditions that start either in the joint itself or in the bursae or the surrounding ligaments. Much more rarely, gout, psuedogout, or infection can be present.

The decision chart indicates that you won't have to see the doctor for most shoulder problems. However, be rather careful with the shoulder. If your home treatment is not progressing well, don't put off the doctor visit too long or you may end with a permanently stiff shoulder and a long series of treatments to loosen it up.

Home Treatment

Treatment involves resting the sore area in combination with exercise to prevent adhesions and stiffness. It's the old problem of rest versus exercise, and you need both in carefully considered amounts.

Rest means take it easy and listen to the pain message. Try not to do things that hurt or that make the pain worse the next day. Avoid the activity that started the whole thing. Common sense will tell you what to do.

Better rest can be obtained with a sling. To fashion a sling, you need two big safety pins and a square piece of cloth two to three feet on a side. Fold the cloth diagonally to make a triangle. Put your forearm across the middle of the triangle with your wrist at the right-angle corner. Have a helper tie or pin the free ends of the triangle behind your neck. Pin up the triangular cravat around the elbow as if you are wrapping a package. This simple sling is the most important treatment for everything from a broken shoulder to acute calcific tendonitis. Wear it all the time for the first few days, then decrease use as the pain subsides.

Exercise absolutely must be done, but it must be "passive." You are not trying to build strength but to keep things loose. Work the shoulder through its normal motion in all direc-

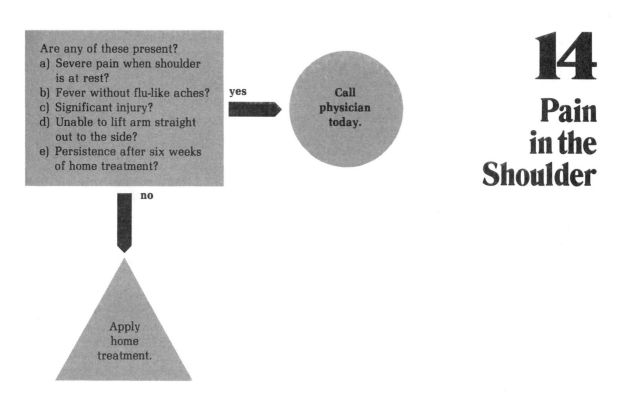

Are any of these present?
a) Severe pain when shoulder is at rest?
b) Fever without flu-like aches?
c) Significant injury?
d) Unable to lift arm straight out to the side?
e) Persistence after six weeks of home treatment?

yes

Call physician today.

no

Apply home treatment.

14
Pain in the Shoulder

tions (or as close to that goal as you can come without too much discomfort) several times each day. Start with "pendulum swings," either dangling your bad arm off the bed or leaning over so that it can hang like a pendulum. Swing it around in little circles and let the circles enlarge. As you get better, you can do this exercise out at the side, where it eventually becomes an "airplane propeller." Try the gentle hand clap—first in front of your chest, then over your head, then behind your back, then repeat. To note your progress, do "wall climbing." Here, you stand sideways to a wall about two feet distant and, with arm straight, walk your fingers up the wall. See how high you can get without too much pain. Make a mark—and try to beat it each day.

Aspirin or acetaminophen may be used to decrease pain, but stay free of major pain-killers. If your doctor has prescribed anti-inflammatory drugs, be sure that you are taking them exactly as prescribed.

What to Expect at the Doctor's Office

The doctor will examine the shoulder and its range of motion. X-rays may be taken and may show calcium deposits, but this is neither good nor bad and doesn't change the treatment. You may be given an anti-inflammatory drug. You should be instructed in exercises and you should set up a future appointment to make sure things are going well. If you don't do the exercises or if the doctor isn't familiar with them, you may be sent to a physical therapist for instruction or treatment. The shoulder may be injected with a steroid—this often helps. In severe, late cases, the joint may be "mobilized under anesthesia" to loosen it up. This rather primitive approach is surprisingly useful. Surgery is not terribly useful in most instances; for example, calcium removal is often unsuccessful. The artificial shoulder joint appears promising, but is still experimental.

15

Pain in the Elbow

The elbow is really two closely related joints. One is a simple hinge joint that operates from straight to about 150° of flexion. The second allows the forearm to twist. The first action allows us to eat, and the second is required to eat soup. Several structures around the elbow may give trouble. Over the point of the elbow is the olecranon bursa, a frequent location for bursitis. On the inside and outside of the elbow are bony bumps to which the muscles attach. These are frequent sites of tendinitis; for example, tennis elbow is a tendinitis on the outside bump. The joint space can be the location of infection or gout; these conditions will cause the part to hurt even though it is not being moved. Young children, usually after being swung by their arms by their parents, sometimes suffer a kind of dislocation. The elbow is exposed enough so that fracture is not uncommon. This injury can be messy to treat because the bones that usually break are right at the joint.

Home Treatment

Apply rest combined with exercises to prevent stiffness. If you know the cause of the problem, stop doing it. For example, a tennis elbow is caused by a bad, jerky backhand, which puts extra strain where the forearm muscle joins the bone. You can stop tennis for a while and you can later take some lessons to improve that stroke. For tennis elbow, an elastic strap over the upper forearm (available at tennis shops) will take some tension off the sore tendon.

Listen for the pain message and let it tell you what not to do. Avoid activities that make it worse either right away or the next day. Remember that you have to let the inflammation subside and the part heal; at least six weeks are required to build full strength. To avoid reinjury, your activity must be below the level that would tear the weakened tendon.

Avoid strong painkillers as they get in the way of your reception of the pain message. Aspirin or acetaminophen are all right, but they won't help you too much.

Rest means take it easy with the elbow. The sling (triangular cravat) described in problem 14 is the best way to rest it. Wear the sling every day for at least a few days; it will rest the elbow and will keep you from using it.

Exercise starts from day one. As with the shoulder, we don't want to build strength, we just want to keep the joint loose so that adhesions and stiffness do not result. The most likely deformity is inability to straighten the arm, so we want to pay particular attention to that motion. Exercise is passive and very simple. Straighten the arm out. Let it hang by your side. Flex it and let it straighten out again. Do this at least ten times twice a day, but don't force too hard at first. If the elbow is really tight, exercise in the shower with warm water running on the elbow. Then, twist the forearm. Start with your arm extended outward, palm facing the floor, then turn your palm upward to face the ceiling. Repeat ten times, twice a day. As you get better, do the exercises faster and force them a little harder. But don't force all the way. As soon as you feel the beginning of pain, back off.

Remember to take anti-inflammatory drugs just as prescribed. If you have been lazy and skipped some doses, that might just be the cause of your flare-up.

What to Expect at the Doctor's Office

The doctor will examine the elbow and its motion. X-rays are likely if you have had an injury, but are of little value otherwise. If the elbow is swollen, fluid may be withdrawn through a needle. This is quick, easy, and pretty safe, and can give good information about gout or infection. You may be given a nonsteroidal anti-inflammatory drug or, if you are already taking one, the dosage may be increased. Injection with a corticosteroid can sometimes be helpful if the problem is synovitis

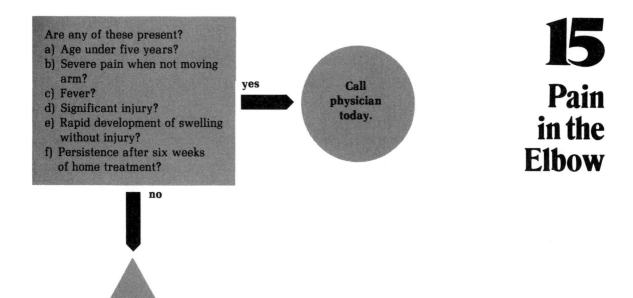

Are any of these present?
a) Age under five years?
b) Severe pain when not moving arm?
c) Fever?
d) Significant injury?
e) Rapid development of swelling without injury?
f) Persistence after six weeks of home treatment?

yes → Call physician today.

no ↓ Apply home treatment.

in the joint space; it has some hazard if the injection is around a tendon, because the tendon can be weakened. At any rate, you shouldn't have more than an occasional injection. Elbows have been destroyed in athletes by repeated injection combined with continuing the activity that caused the problem. Surgery is rarely needed unless there is a fracture, in which case the bones may need to be surgically set and a pin may need to be placed. You may be sent to a physical therapist, but it is usually better for you to do your own exercises regularly rather than relying on professional treatment just three times a week.

16

Pain in the Wrist

The wrist is an unusual joint because stiffness or even fusion causes relatively little difficulty, while lack of stability can pose real problems. The wrist provides the platform from which the fine motions of the fingers operate; it is essential that this platform be stable. The eight wrist bones form a rather crude joint that is very limited in motion compared with, say, the shoulder, but which is strong and stable. Almost no regular human activities require the wrist to be bent all the way back or all the way forward, and the fingers don't operate as well when the wrist is fully flexed or fully extended.

The wrist platform works best when the wrist is bent upward just a little. To illustrate this position, make a fist and put your thumb in the middle of your fist. Looking down your arm, the thumb should be on an imaginary line going straight down the middle of your forearm. Thus, any item in your grasp, if the wrist is in proper position, can be pulled or pushed in the most efficient manner.

The wrist can be affected by synovitis, as in rheumatoid arthritis, can be infected, or can be the site of gout or pseudogout. With injury, the wrist may be sprained or the forearm bones may break just above the wrist, the *Colles fracture*. With gonorrhea, the back of the wrist may be inflamed and wiggling the fingers may be painful. This *tenosynovitis* of the wrist may occur together with another clue to VD, a small red skin mark with a little blister in the center.

The *carpal-tunnel syndrome* can cause pain at the wrist. In addition, it can cause pains to shoot down into the fingers or up into the forearm. Usually there is a numb feeling in the fingers, as if they were asleep. In this syndrome, the median nerve is trapped and squeezed as it passes through the fibrous carpal tunnel in the front of the wrist. Usually the squeezing results from too much inflammatory tissue. The cause can be tennis playing, a blow to the front of the wrist, canoe paddling, rheumatoid arthritis, or a lot of other problems. You can diagnose this syndrome pretty well yourself. The numbness in the fingers will not involve the little finger and often will not involve the half of the ring finger nearest the little finger. If you tap with a finger on the front of the wrist, you may get a sudden tingling in the fingers similar to the feeling of hitting your "funny bone." Tingling and pain may be worse at night or when the wrists are cocked down.

Home Treatment.

A splint is splendid. Since stability is essential and loss of motion is not as serious in the wrist as in other joints, the treatment strategy is a little different. Exercises to increase the motion of the joint are not as important. The strategy is to rest the joint in the position of best function. Wrist splints are available at hospital supply stores and some drugstores. Any that fit you are probably all right. The splint will be of plastic or aluminum and the hand rest will cock your wrist back just a bit. You can put a cloth sleeve around the splint to make it more comfortable against your skin and wrap the splint and your arm gently with an elastic bandage to keep it in place. That's all there is to it. Wear it all the time for a few days, then just at night for a few weeks. This simple treatment is all that is required for most wrist flare-ups. Even the carpal-tunnel syndrome is initially treated by splinting. But, since nerve damage is potentially serious, give your doctor a call if you seem to have this syndrome and discuss your plan.

No major pain medication should be necessary; aspirin and similar-strength medications are all right, but probably won't help too much. If you are taking a prescribed anti-inflammatory drug, be certain that you are taking it just as directed; sometimes a flare-up is simply due to inadequate medication.

If you know what triggered the pain, work out a way to avoid that activity. Common sense means listening to the pain message.

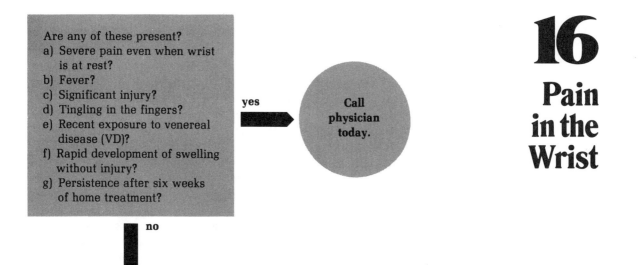

Are any of these present?
a) Severe pain even when wrist is at rest?
b) Fever?
c) Significant injury?
d) Tingling in the fingers?
e) Recent exposure to venereal disease (VD)?
f) Rapid development of swelling without injury?
g) Persistence after six weeks of home treatment?

yes → Call physician today.

no → Apply home treatment.

16
Pain in the Wrist

What to Expect at the Doctor's Office

Examination of the sore wrist followed by advice similar to that above can be expected. X-rays may be required, but rarely. Anti-inflammatory drugs may be prescribed. Injection with a steroid may be performed on occasion, and is likely if a carpal-tunnel syndrome has not responded to splinting. Surgery of several different kinds is available and one or another procedure may be recommended, depending on your problem. The carpal-tunnel nerve compression may be surgically released. In rheumatoid arthritis, the synovial tissue on the back of the hand may be removed to protect the tendons that run through the inflamed area. The wrist may be casted or fused. Rarely, removal of the ends of the forearm bones will help prevent further damage.

17

Pain in the Fingers

Each hand has fourteen finger joints, each of which acts like a small hinge. Because the joints are small, they are operated by muscles in the forearm that control the joints by an intricate system of small slings for the tendon leaders. The small size and complicated arrangements mean that any inflammation or damage to the joint is likely to result in some stiffness and lost motion, as even a small adhesion will limit motion.

So, you shouldn't expect that a problem with a small finger joint will resolve completely. Even after healing is complete, some left-over stiffness and occasional twinges of discomfort are likely. Unrealistically high expectations lead to feelings that you did something wrong or that the doctor was no good. In fact, almost all of us have a few fingers that have been injured and remain a bit crooked or stiff. The hand functions very well with such deformities; fingers need not open fully or close completely to be perfectly functional.

These small joints are very seldom the location for gout or bacterial infection. But in rheumatoid arthritis, lupus, and other forms of synovitis, the finger joints are often the most affected of any joints. Virus arthritis, drug allergies, and serum sickness all commonly affect the small finger joints. Osteoarthritis frequently causes knobby swelling of the most distant joints of the fingers. Rheumatoid arthritis usually concentrates on the middle joints (PIP) and the joints at the near end of the fingers (MCP). Scleroderma can cause loss of motion by tightening of the skin. Sprains, strains, and small fractures are common.

Home Treatment

Listen to the pain message and avoid activities that cause or aggravate pain. Rest the finger joints so that they can heal, but use gentle stretching exercises to keep them limber and maintain motion. You can't cast the fingers very well and splints tend to leave stiff joints behind, so the key to managing your finger arthritis is to use common sense.

With a bit of ingenuity, you can find a less stressful way to do almost any activity that puts stress on the joints. Since everyone's activities are a bit different, you'll have to invent these new ways yourself. Here are a few hints to get you going. A big handle can be gripped with less strain than a small handle, so wrapping pens, knives, and other similar objects with tape or putting a sponge-rubber handle over the original handle can protect the grip. Lift smaller loads. Make more trips. Plan ahead rather than blundering through an activity. Let others open the car door for you. Get power steering or a very light car. Use a gripper for opening tough jar lids or stop buying products that come in hard-to-open jars. When opening a tough lid, apply friction pressure on the top of the lid with your palm and twist with your whole hand, not your grip. Cultivate ingenious friends who are handy at making little gadgets to help you. Don't put heavy objects too high or too low. Organize your kitchen, workshop, study, and bedroom.

Stretch the joints gently twice a day to maintain motion. Straighten the hand out against the tabletop. Make a fist and then cock the wrist to increase the stretch. Use one hand to move each finger of the other hand through full flexing to straight out. Don't force, but stretch just to the edge of discomfort. If the motion of a joint is normal, one repetition is enough, but if the motion is limited, do ten repetitions. Warming the hands in warm water before stretching may help you get more motion.

Don't use strong pain medications; they mask the pain so that you may overdo an activity or an exercise. Be sure that you take prescribed medication for inflammation just exactly as instructed. Good hand function is important and you want to pay close attention to treatment.

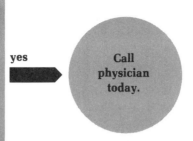

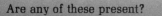

Are any of these present?
a) Severe pain when fingers are at rest?
b) Fingers cannot be straightened out?
c) Significant injury?
d) Numbness or tingling in the fingers?
e) Persistence after six weeks of home treatment?

yes → Call physician today.

no

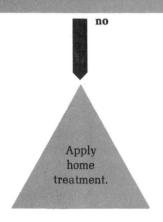

Apply home treatment.

What to Expect at the Doctor's Office

The doctor will examine your hands and their motions. Sometimes, an X-ray is taken, but usually not more often than every two years. An increase in anti-inflammatory medications may be needed. Rarely, injection of a particularly bad joint is helpful, but this is less effective with small joints than with large ones. Surgery is also less effective with small joints and isn't indicated often. Surgery, such as placement of plastic joints or removal of inflamed tissue, usually makes the hand look more normal and sometimes decreases the pain, but the hand often doesn't work much better than it did before the operation.

18

Pain at Night

Night pain is really an indication of the severity of pain. Usually, pain will decrease at night as the body diminishes its sensation input for sleep and becomes less active. Typically, a patient with arthritis may have occasional night pains when changing position, but will be free of serious discomfort for most of the night. While it may seem that sleep is lost by these brief episodes, the body gets plenty of sleep and no serious problem is present.

Most people overestimate the magnitude of a sleeping problem. Unless the sleeping time totals less than four hours, the body is very good at substituting quality for quantity. The drive to sleep is overwhelming and the truly tired person will sleep under the most adverse circumstances. Once in a great while, a vicious cycle occurs in which pain prevents sleep, fatigue prevents rational approaches to problems during the day, depression aggravates pain, and sleep is even more disturbed by pain and depression. The hints given here can help with most of these problems.

Home Treatment

Have a comfortable bed. Usually a moderately firm mattress of good quality is the best choice. A waterbed, which supports the weight of the body evenly and can be kept quite warm, is very successful for some people with arthritis, while others never can get used to the thing. Pillows can be used here and there to increase comfort. For example, they can be placed on the sides to limit turning, under the neck, under the low back, or below the feet to keep the covers off the feet. Be careful not to use a pillow under the knees if there is any problem

with the knees or hips, as a stiff contracture can result.

Don't go to bed early to try to ensure enough sleep. Wait until you're tired. You want your body so ready to sleep that it suppresses painful signals from the nerves.

Beware of sedatives and sleeping pills. These give the wrong kind of sleep, cause rebound depression in some people, tend to be habit forming, and only very rarely help solve sleeping problems.

Beware also of painkilling drugs. These do not affect the arthritis but only suppress the symptoms, and the symptom of night pain is one that should be listened to. The body has mechanisms for adjusting to long-term pain and many doctors feel that pain medications interfere with normal adaptation to pain.

The sleeping partner is important. A restless partner may make twin beds advisable. On the other hand, sexual relations at bedtime encourage good relaxation and healthy sleep.

Be sure to take your anti-inflammatory drugs as prescribed. If your doctor has encouraged you to adjust your own doses, try to increase the number of times each day that you take the medication and to be sure that you have a dose at bedtime. Setting the alarm so as to take another dose in the middle of the night may be worthwhile.

What to Expect at the Doctor's Office

The complaint of night pain is a signal to your doctor that your arthritis needs some attention. Examination, tests, even X-rays may be required. A new treatment program may be developed, emphasizing more powerful anti-inflammatory medicines. Most experienced doctors will be cautious with pain medication and sedatives and will try to deal with the underlying problem.

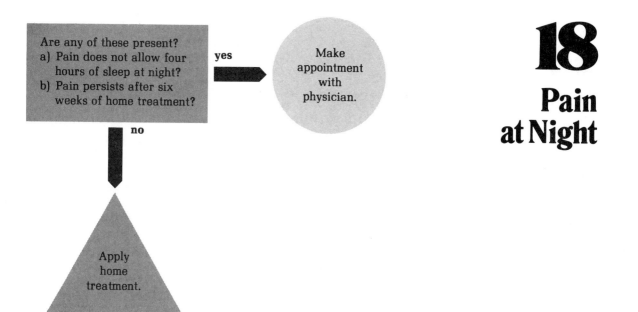

Are any of these present?
a) Pain does not allow four hours of sleep at night?
b) Pain persists after six weeks of home treatment?

yes → Make appointment with physician.

no ↓

Apply home treatment.

18

Pain at Night

19

Pain after Exercise

Quite simply, if you are getting pain after exercise, your body is telling you not to do the activity that caused the pain. The pain message is your most important ally as you fight your arthritis. Listen to it.

Underlying this problem is a less simple paradox. To get better, you have to increase your exercise, and this inevitably will trigger at least a few episodes of increased pain. This is not a message to eliminate the exercise program! Rather, it is a suggestion from your body to proceed more carefully with your planned exercise progression. So, don't be discouraged by pain after exercise. Listen to it and work with it.

Discomfort immediately after exercise is common with mechanical problems such as strains, fractures, or degenerated cartilage. Inflammatory conditions such as synovitis or attachment arthritis often get better with movement, while mechanical problems get worse. The day after the exercise, almost any form of arthritis or rheumatism may feel worse.

You don't need the doctor unless signs of severe injury or nerve damage are present or unless the problem continues to bother you quite a bit for quite a while. This problem is a signal to review your home exercise program.

Home Treatment

Almost always, pain indicates that you have disregarded one of the principles of a sound exercise program. Let's review them.

Exercise should not make you hurt very much. Don't try to exercise through pain. If you hurt after exercise, that exercise is a bit too much for you right now.

Exercise programs should be daily. The weekend warrior is not going to become fit or able, will have reinjuries, and will experience increased pain and stiffness on Mondays.

Exercise programs should be gently graded. No day's activity should be more than a 10 percent increase over the previous day's activity. Slow and steady progression is essential to success.

Exercise programs should emphasize smooth actions, as with swimming, walking, or bicycling, until good conditioning is achieved. Jerky exercises with incompletely trained muscles are likely to result in reinjury.

Exercise programs should emphasize suppleness and muscle tone, not absolute strength. The stress of lifting heavy objects, squeezing balls, and so forth is likely to damage an already injured joint. Swimming easily is the perfect exercise.

Exercise should be preceded by a warm-up period in which the joints, ligaments, and muscles are stretched gently. The parts to be used should be physically warm; on a cold day, wear warm-up clothing.

Exercise programs are in addition to, not instead of, prescribed medications. Adherence to prescribed medication programs, particularly with anti-inflammatory drugs, may be essential to your success with exercise.

Now, review your plan, revise it if necessary, and get on with it.

What to Expect at the Doctor's Office

The physician will reinforce the concepts reviewed above. If you have trouble figuring out how to apply the principles, you may be referred to a physical therapist. Anti-inflammatory medication might be increased. Your understanding of the exercise program and of the patience required to recondition your body are essential. Older people are likely to think that serious exercise programs are for the young. This is absolutely not so—the principles of conditioning apply to all ages. You won't get as well as you might unless you persevere in your exercise program.

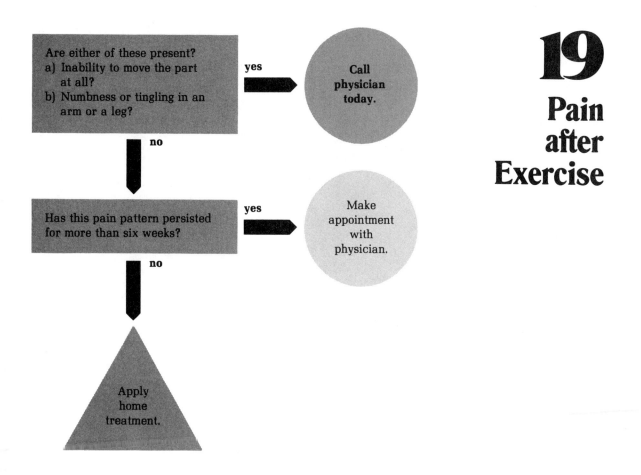

Are either of these present?
a) Inability to move the part at all?
b) Numbness or tingling in an arm or a leg?

yes → Call physician today.

no

Has this pain pattern persisted for more than six weeks?

yes → Make appointment with physician.

no

Apply home treatment.

19
Pain after Exercise

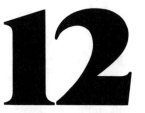

Problems Usually
Caused by Medications

20

Skin
Rash

Allergy is a strong signal to stop the offending medicine. Skin rash and asthmatic attacks are the most common drug allergies, and only skin rash is common with drugs used for arthritis. Still, if you think that wheezing or difficulty in breathing might be due to a drug, then you should call your doctor without delay.

Any new skin rash while on any medication should raise suspicion in your mind. Any drug can cause a rash, and even the "inert" ingredients in tablets have been found to cause rashes. A drug rash can become severe if the drug is continued after the rash has been noticed. So, call the doctor before taking any more tablets.

Some drugs are more likely to cause rash than are others. In arthritis patients, penicillin or ampicillin are the most frequent rash producers. Although they are not drugs used for treating arthritis very often, they are frequently given to arthritis patients for other reasons. Other antibiotics, including sulfa, are often implicated. Drug-induced lupus may be caused by procaine amide, isoniazid (INH), hydralazine, and other drugs. Allopurinol causes skin rash in up to 5 percent of persons taking this drug. Toxic reactions to gold and penicillamine may involve skin rash, often with mouth ulcers as well.

On the other hand, some drugs are pretty unlikely to cause rash. Aspirin, acetaminophen (Tylenol), OH-chloroquine (Plaquenil), colchicine, and prednisone hardly ever cause a rash.

A drug rash is usually fairly widespread over the trunk and arms. It may be most severe in the body creases. It usually itches and is usually red in color. There may or may not be fever with it.

Some rashes are obviously the disease and not the drug—for example, the sharply defined "butterfly" rash over the nose and cheeks seen in lupus, the small black sores at the corners of the nails in rheumatoid arthritis, or the lilac-colored knuckles and eyelids in dermatomyositis. Other disease-caused rashes include the occasional "fried egg" blister on a red base in gonococcal arthritis, the rapidly disappearing rash on the trunk in juvenile arthritis, scaling patches on the soles in Reiter's syndrome, and painful blisters in one part of the body with complicating "shingles." Pitted nails and scaling patches are characteristic of psoriatic arthritis.

Home Treatment

The easiest rash of all to cure is a drug rash. Usually it will be very much better within two days; all you do is stop the drug after talking with your doctor, and wait. If the rash itches a lot, a warm bath with two tablespoons of baking soda in it can help. If the rash persists, check again with your doctor. Tell your doctor about any drug rash you may have had; you may need new medication or perhaps some tests for allergic damage to other organs.

What to Expect at the Doctor's Office

The drug will be stopped if there is a reasonable suspicion that it is causing the rash. If possible, the doctor will keep you off all drugs for a while; often a suspected allergic reaction is a good chance to review the entire treatment program. New drugs, with different chemical formulas so that they will not "cross-react," may be prescribed. Drugs may be reintroduced carefully one at a time if several are suspected. Blood tests for liver or kidney damage may be requested.

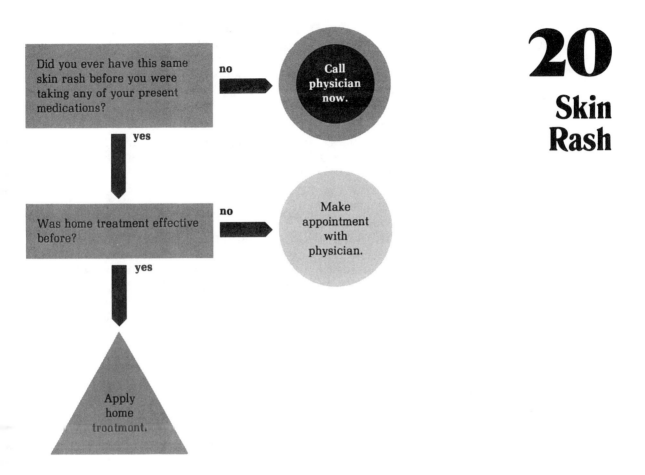

Did you ever have this same skin rash before you were taking any of your present medications?

no → Call physician now.

yes ↓

Was home treatment effective before?

no → Make appointment with physician.

yes ↓

Apply home treatment.

21

Nausea or Vomiting

Nausea and vomiting have a whole host of causes. Of course there is the flu. Or it may be ulcers, food poisoning, gall-bladder problems, or motion sickness. On the other hand, if you're taking a drug for arthritis and have nausea or vomiting, chances are that the drug is responsible.

Most stomach problems from drugs are due to direct irritation of the stomach lining. If you look in the stomach with a gastroscope, you may see an area of gastritis with the pill sitting in the middle of the inflamed area. Some of the drugs that can cause gastritis also can cause nausea by certain effects on the brain, but almost always the direct irritation is the major problem. Direct irritant drugs include aspirin, Indocin, Motrin, Nalfon, Naprosyn, Tolectin, Butazolidine, and some others.

Some other drugs wreak havoc on your GI tract differently. Prednisone and other steroids seem to increase the acid in the stomach while decreasing the mucus layer that protects the stomach lining. Colchicine usually causes diarrhea, but a few patients experience nausea as well. Gold salts and penicillamine sometimes cause ulcers in the mouth or stomach wall which are not due to direct toxicity, but can result in nausea or vomiting.

Finally, some powerful immunosuppressant drugs seem to cause nausea by interfering with cell division and cell repair in the stomach and small intestine. These drugs include Imuran, Cytoxan, methotrexate, and chlorambucil.

Some drugs are generally pretty safe for the stomach. Acetaminophen and hydroxychloroquine (Plaquenil) are examples.

Home treatment works best for the direct irritant drugs. This side effect is a double problem; you don't want to lose the use of a good drug because of a minor side effect, but you also don't want the problem to become major. The best practice is to try home treatment first (it will usually work). If it fails, ask your doctor for some more hints. Finally, switch medications if your stomach is just too sensitive. Good judgment is needed to know when to stop a drug that is causing nausea or stomach pain. Check with your doctor if you aren't sure what to do.

Home Treatment

If your doctor has told you to take the suspected drug only if you need it, try stopping the drug for a few days and start over with a more comfortable stomach. If your doctor wants you to take the medicine regularly, then try these tricks. Space the same dose out through the day. For example, instead of two tablets every four hours, try one tablet every two hours. Take at least an eight-ounce glass of water with each dose to dilute the chemical in the stomach. Take the drug after meals, when the food in the stomach will help protect the stomach lining. Or, take one ounce of a liquid antacid (such as Maalox, Gelusil, or Riopan) a few minutes before you take the medication dose.

If these don't work, try around-the-clock buffering. Eat six small meals a day instead of three big ones. Keep something in the stomach each hour when awake; if this is not a meal, then make it an ounce of antacid. Set the alarm to go off during the night, take some antacid, and then reset the alarm for a few hours later. Check with the doctor if you don't seem to be making good progress; this regimen should make you more comfortable in just a couple of days.

Remember that side effects are to be expected from drugs. We just have to keep them at the level of minor annoyances, not major problems.

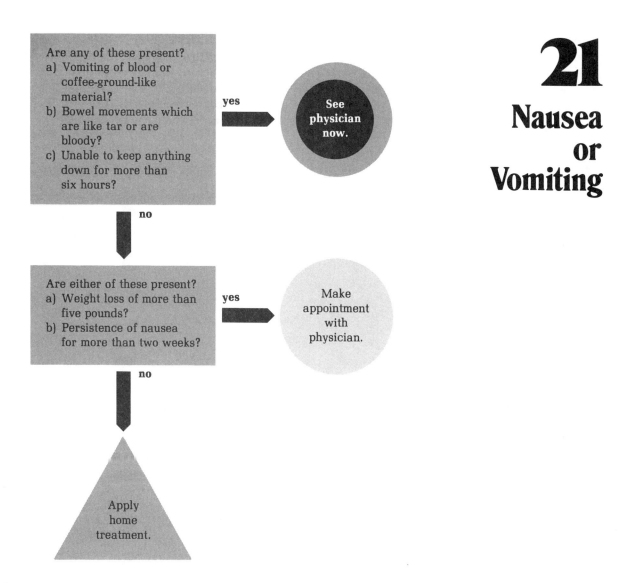

Are any of these present?
a) Vomiting of blood or coffee-ground-like material?
b) Bowel movements which are like tar or are bloody?
c) Unable to keep anything down for more than six hours?

yes → See physician now.

no ↓

Are either of these present?
a) Weight loss of more than five pounds?
b) Persistence of nausea for more than two weeks?

yes → Make appointment with physician.

no ↓

Apply home treatment.

What to Expect at the Doctor's Office

The doctor will ask some questions and may have some further suggestions. If the problem is major, you may have to have a gastroscopy (interior examination of the stomach) or an X-ray of the stomach. Usually, however, it is simpler just to stop the drug. Your doctor will try to suggest a medication that will cause less irritation and do the same job for your arthritis.

22

Ringing in the Ears

Aspirin is the most likely cause of this problem. The second most likely cause is aspirin. So is the third. Possibly, other anti-inflammatory drugs cause *tinnitus*, which is the medical word for "ringing in the ears," but aspirin is overwhelmingly the major cause.

This is a warning sign of aspirin toxicity. It means that the aspirin level in your blood is approaching the upper margin of safety. If you take more aspirin, the sequence of events is something like this. The first ringing is mild and is noticed about one to two hours after the last dose. Then the ringing becomes louder and constant. Hearing begins to decrease and the ringing may seem to improve simply because you can't hear it as well. You experience shortness of breath and begin to breathe hard and fast. You now have moderately severe aspirin toxicity.

Serious aspirin toxicity is rare in adults. It is more frequently seen in children who manage to get into the "child-proof" bottles. Don't be frightened by the sequence above; aspirin remains one of our safest medications. All drugs are subject to overuse and aspirin is no exception.

When you stop the aspirin, the aspirin level in your blood begins to decrease and will decline slowly over several days. As it goes down, the sequence will reverse. Damage is not permanent, except for very rare hearing damage in very severe cases. If you had a damaged liver before the episode, the aspirin may remain in your blood even longer, since the liver acts to remove the aspirin from the body. If you are short of breath, call the doctor and discuss the situation. It is probably due to the aspirin and will go away within the day, but it could always be something else.

For most people, about 16 to 20 tablets a day are required to get the blood level high enough for the ears to ring. An occasional patient reports it at a lower level, but such instances often reflect patient nervousness rather than true ringing of the ears. Some people don't get ringing before 40 tablets (200 grains) a day; other people get decreased hearing first and don't notice the ringing. If you have a preexisting hearing problem, you should be a bit more careful with aspirin, since you might not get the warning signal of ringing. Be alert for a further decrease in hearing.

Remember, aspirin is in a wide variety of patent medicines. ASA, aspirin, and acetylsalicylic acid all describe the same drug. Anacin, Bufferin, Alka-Selzer, Contac, APC's, Dristan, Midol, and practically every other cold tablet or pain reliever contains aspirin. Exceptions are those medications containing acetaminophen, such as Tylenol.

Home Treatment

Stop all aspirin-containing medication and wait for the ringing to go away. This may take only two hours or it may take two days. Ringing in the ears is *not* a reason to stop the medication permanently. It is merely a signal to use a somewhat lower dose. So, gradually start the medication again and keep to a slightly lower dose. If your ears rang the first time at 16 tablets a day, try 14. If they ring again at 14, try 12. Ringing will be less and arthritis benefit more if you spread the doses out over the whole day as best you can, rather than taking a few large doses of 4 or 5 tablets at once.

Ringing in the ears is a good sign. It means that your body absorbs the aspirin well and that you can get good blood levels in order to decrease the inflammation. You are likely to get a good result from your aspirin treatment after the dose is adjusted appropriately.

What to Expect at the Doctor's Office

The advice above will be repeated by your physician. If your problem is severe, blood tests of liver and kidney function may be done. Doctors are encouraged by this complaint, because it indicates a patient who can be counted on to take a prescribed medication. Ringing in the ears happens to the "best" patients.

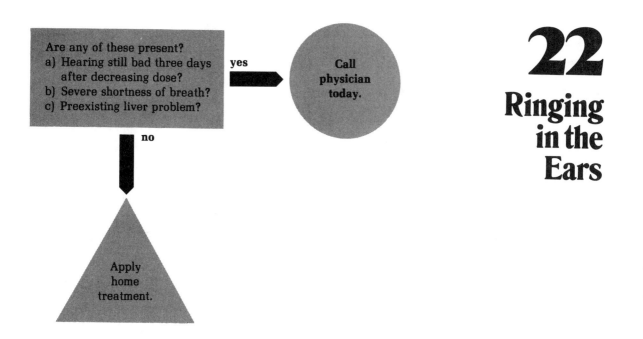

Are any of these present?
a) Hearing still bad three days
   after decreasing dose?
b) Severe shortness of breath?
c) Preexisting liver problem?

yes

Call
physician
today.

no

Apply
home
treatment.

22

**Ringing
in the
Ears**

23

Dizziness
or
Headache

These problems have a lot of different possible causes and you may want to check out the more general discussion that appears in *Take Care of Yourself* (Addison-Wesley, 1978). Here, we want to make the point that these problems can be the side effects of drugs given for arthritis. You should always be ready to suspect any drug of anything, but there are certain circumstances in which dizziness or headache are most likely to be drug related.

Aspirin in high doses of 12 or more tablets daily can cause dizziness and light-headedness in addition to the symptoms listed in problem 22.

Indomethacin (Indocin) is the most notorious of arthritis drugs with regard to these problems. Severe headaches, dizziness, and feelings of detachment are common, particularly in the first few weeks of taking the medication. Usually, but not always, this problem gets better after you have taken the indomethacin for a while.

Less frequently, other anti-inflammatory drugs can cause these problems.

Painkillers, including codeine, Percodan, Darvon, and Talwin, can cause dizziness and unusual "drugged" mental sensations, but do not cause head pain.

Home Treatment

Decrease or stop taking the drug after talking with your doctor. Wait and see if the problem diminishes over a short period, usually less than 24 hours. If the dizziness persists, the drug probably is not responsible and you should think through the problem again. If in doubt, discuss the problem with your doctor.

What to Expect at the Doctor's Office

These problems are difficult for the doctor. The most problematical question is how far to proceed with investigations and tests that usually don't reveal anything and, even if they do identify an abnormality, don't suggest a good treatment. Often these problems persist for some time on and off, but still don't amount to anything major.

In addition to drug causes, nervousness or anxiety, low blood pressure, vertigo, virus, tension, depression, brain tumor, stroke, ear infection, or a hundred other possible causes may be to blame. Skull X-rays usually do not help in a diagnosis. Brain-wave tests, arteriograms, and blood tests usually aren't much help either. So, the decisions are difficult. You often can help by not pushing the doctor to do more and more. Just how much investigation is appropriate depends on how long you have had the problem, how much of a problem it poses in your daily life, and what other problems you are having at the same time.

210

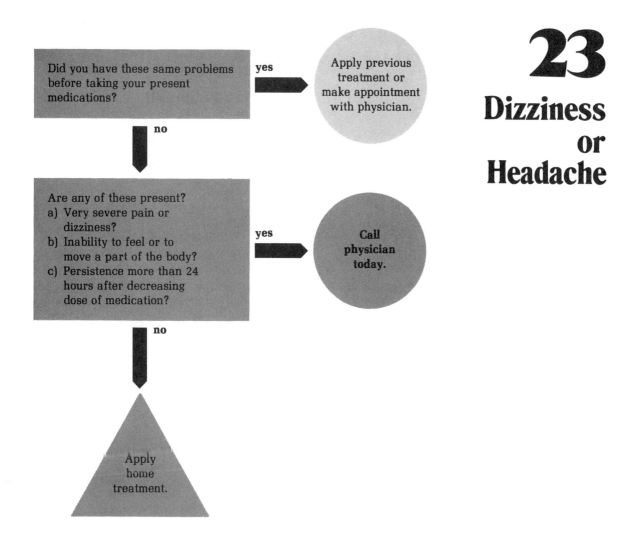

Did you have these same problems before taking your present medications?

yes → Apply previous treatment or make appointment with physician.

no ↓

Are any of these present?
a) Very severe pain or dizziness?
b) Inability to feel or to move a part of the body?
c) Persistence more than 24 hours after decreasing dose of medication?

yes → Call physician today.

no ↓

Apply home treatment.

23
Dizziness
or
Headache

13

Problems Getting Around

24

Difficulty Getting Dressed

The rest of the problem discussions in this section relate to daily living. Arthritis can limit your everyday activities, either for the short term or the long term. These limitations are especially frustrating, because we take our ability to perform these simple tasks for granted. The frustration sometimes leads to withdrawal rather than to confronting and dealing with the problem. Usually these problems are readily solved without professional help. Developing your own solutions can be a source of real satisfaction. If your arthritis is sufficiently severe to affect your daily life, take pride in finding ways to meet the challenge. A few techniques are suggested here, but you will have to adapt and invent to find your best solutions.

Problems with dressing are usually related to the fine finger movements needed to fasten small buttons, the shoulder action necessary to get clothes over the head or to fasten garments behind the back, or the difficulty in reaching the feet to put on trousers, shoes, or socks. Other people may have trouble pulling open a dresser drawer or getting to the dresser.

While patients with rheumatoid arthritis most frequently have problems of this kind, a young man with low back pain or a child with a broken elbow faces the same challenges for a shorter time.

Home Treatment

The idea is to make everything as easy as possible. Put the dresser near the bed. Use a dresser of light-weight wood with small, well-lubricated drawers. Replace small knobs with big handles.

Select clothes that are easy to put on: slip-on shoes, front-fastening garments, zippers with big ring pulls, wrap-around robes, clothes with Velcro fasteners, clip-on ties, stretch belts that hook rather than buckle.

Get a friend—or several. A spouse is fine, or a friend with whom you can exchange tasks, each of you doing what you are good at. A friendly handyperson and someone who can use a sewing machine, if you cannot, can be very helpful. Velcro, a marvelous material that sticks to itself simply by applying slight pressure and pulls apart just as easily, can be a wonderful replacement for buttons, shoelaces, belts, bra hooks, and other fastenings. You can sew it on everything. The handyperson can make some of the gadgets you may need.

Get gadgets. A long-handled shoehorn, garter snaps or spring clothespins on a piece of tape for helping to put on socks, and a closet hook on the end of a dowel to extend your reach can make life much simpler. Other suggestions are a valet stand to hold your shirt while you put an arm through, a wire buttonhook for small buttons, and a collar extender loop to make buttoning that top collar button easier.

What to Expect from the Health Professional

Occupational therapists are trained to help you with this kind of problem. The key word is "adaptive"; the therapist will suggest ways in which you can adapt to your disability. The therapist will also know the sources in your area for gadgets and appliances. Every patient with a long-term arthritis problem should purchase the handbook *Self-Help Manual* from the Arthritis Foundation. It is a gold mine of hints, pictures, and sources for materials.

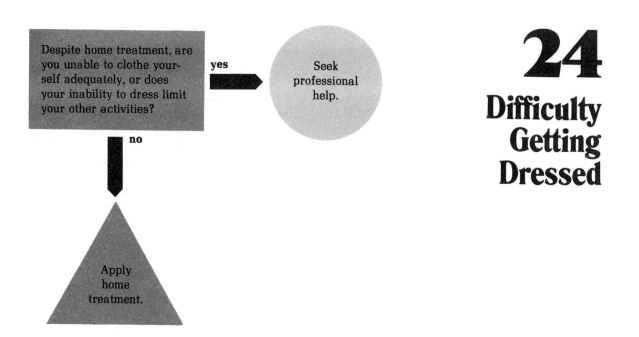

Despite home treatment, are you unable to clothe yourself adequately, or does your inability to dress limit your other activities?

yes → Seek professional help.

no ↓

Apply home treatment.

24
Difficulty Getting Dressed

25

Problems Using the Toilet

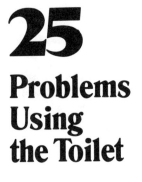

Dignity is a crucial part of the problem here, since we usually don't feel comfortable asking another person to help us with our eliminations. So, this problem very often goes unmentioned. However, with a few fairly simple measures, a lot of difficulty can be avoided.

Remember, the idea is to make necessary daily activities as easy as possible. This is a sensible idea for everybody, of course, but if you have a physical limitation, the defects in the way our society is designed suddenly become very obvious. What is merely an annoyance for others is a real nuisance to you. And, if you can save a few seconds (and some energy) at tasks you must repeat many times, the savings become substantial.

The biggest problem is usually the effort involved in getting on and off of the toilet. Muscle weakness in the legs, contractures of the hips, and arthritis of the knees all act to make getting up and down a problem. We discouraged deep knee bends earlier because they stress the knees too much; the action involved in using the toilet is almost the same.

Persons with severe arthritis sometimes have trouble using toilet paper. And a problem with the bowels, whether it is diarrhea or constipation, can make the whole thing more difficult than it need be.

Home Treatment

You need some physical aids. The most important one is a raised toilet seat. In a major remodeling, you can have toilets installed three to five inches higher than standard, or you can simply purchase a raised seat at a hospital supply store. Don't underestimate the importance of the raised seat; many people have trouble visualizing how much it will help until they have tried it.

An armrest unit can be bolted to the toilet bolts and used together with the raised seat. This permits you to use your arms as well as your legs in getting up and down. Alternatively, a safety bar can be installed on the wall. The bar will serve to steady you and to take some of your weight as you stand and sit.

Severely affected persons can use a glider commode to put the toilet in a nearby location, but we don't find too much use for these. Sometimes they encourage a person to be bedbound when he or she could be more active.

For holding toilet paper, your reach can be extended by a variety of different gadgets. You can make tissue holders from knitting needles or coat hangers, or use tongs with plastic tips.

Finally, if money is no object, a bidet can be installed. There are portable bidets that attach to an existing toilet or entire new units can be installed. These use a jet of warm water to cleanse gently. Although relatively rare in the United States, bidets are commonplace in Europe.

Diarrhea or constipation contribute to the problem of using the toilet, either because of increased frequency or increased straining. So, healthy habits (but not obsessions with bowel frequency) are important. A good diet that includes plenty of fruits and vegetables as well as bran and whole-wheat breads should be observed. Exercise regularly and avoid laxatives. If a medication must be taken, use Metamucil—a teaspoonful in a glass of water twice a day. This will increase bulk and stabilize the stool.

What to Expect from the Health Professional

The occupational therapist (OT) may well have some additional hints for you and will know the sources for any purchases you may need. The therapist might visit your home; if so, take advantage of this visit to inquire about hints for the other rooms of your house or apartment.

The social worker may be able to find a source of funds to pay for those things that are too costly for you. Remember that any expendi-

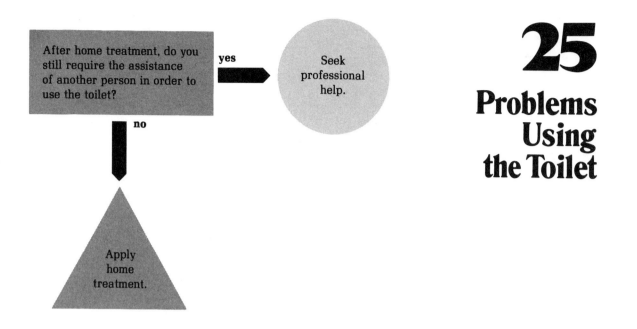

After home treatment, do you still require the assistance of another person in order to use the toilet?

yes → Seek professional help.

no

Apply home treatment.

Problems Using the Toilet

tures you must make to equip your house because of your arthritis are tax deductible; ask your doctor for a prescription for the raised toilet seat, safety bar, or whatever on your next visit. The tax people might want to see it. Your doctor will appreciate your not making a special trip just to obtain such documentation.

26

Problems with Bathing and Hygiene

These activities are closely tied in to how we feel about ourselves, giving them an importance beyond the medical requirement for decent hygiene. We feel helpless and humiliated if we cannot keep ourselves looking clean or if we must worry about the way we may smell—and these worries may cause us to withdraw from social activities. So, these are crucial concerns. The success of other activities may depend on how well we can adapt to problems with bathing, hygiene, and grooming. Some major changes in the home may be necessary for patients with severe arthritis, but the rewards can be dramatic.

Problems usually center around how to get in or out of a tub or shower, or how to hold a toothbrush or comb, or how to reach all parts of the body. The modern house is not very well designed for efficient living and the patient with arthritis needs to live as efficiently as possible. So, you may have to be quite resourceful and do some inventing.

Home Treatment

For a bathtub, mount rails on the wall to help you get in and out safely. Safety rails that mount on the side of the tub are available at hospital supply stores. A suction-cup mat or nonskid tape on the bottom of the tub can prevent you from slipping. A shower is better for many people, but again use the nonskid tape for safety. A telephone-type shower head that moves up and down on a metal rod often helps. Single-lever faucets are easier to manage than old-fashioned ones that require a strong twist to turn on and keep on dripping after you turn them off. Don't use soap dishes or plumbing to hold onto; they can pull out of the wall. A sitting shower is possible if you can't stand for long; use a bath bench with suction cups on the legs. Put the soap in a cloth bag on a string around your neck to eliminate that terrible search for the dropped soap. A shower caddy hanging from the shower head is useful to keep shampoo and brushes close by. A back scrubbing strap can make that chore easy—and it feels good. A bath mitt can help in scrubbing. To dry off, just put on a terry-cloth robe and let it soak up the water.

Put built-up handles on combs, toothbrushes, and hairbrushes. It is much easier to grasp a large handle than a small one. An electric toothbrush can save some effort. If reach is a problem, mount long handles on combs and brushes. You can build up nail clippers with longer wooden handles to make them easier to use. If you mount a nailbrush on suction cups, it will stay put while you scrub. An electric razor is often more manageable than a hand one, and razor holders to improve your grip are available from major manufacturers such as Remington, Sunbeam, and Norelco. Many women prefer a cream-type depilatory for their legs. Sanitary napkins are available with adhesive strips that are easy to fasten. There are even Velcro hair curlers that can be worked with one hand. You won't need to make use of all of these tricks, of course, but they are included to give you an idea of the many ways in which you can simplify an essential everyday activity.

What to Expect from the Health Professional

The occupational therapist can suggest additional ideas and will know where to obtain needed gadgets. The social worker can sometimes help in obtaining funds or in finding used equipment. Remember that devices required for your arthritis can be tax deductible, which decreases the cost to you. These expenditures are worth the cost.

The *Self-Help Manual for Arthritis Patients*, available from the Arthritis Foundation at nominal cost, has lots of additional suggestions.

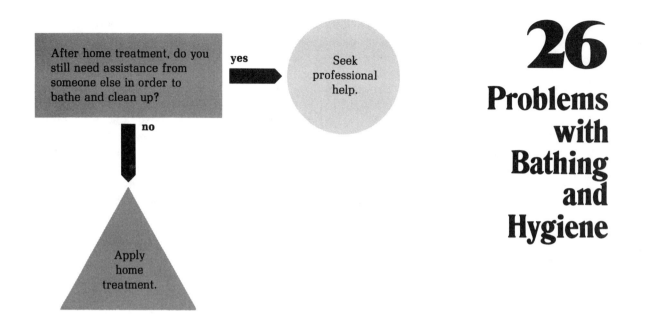

After home treatment, do you still need assistance from someone else in order to bathe and clean up?

yes

Seek professional help.

no

Apply home treatment.

26
Problems with Bathing and Hygiene

27

Difficulty Turning Handles and Opening Doors

When you have arthritis, the world can sometimes seem like an unfriendly place. Design for style rather than for function makes many things difficult even if you have a good thumb and a strong grip. And if you don't, you're in trouble.

Some of these design features are really totally unnecessary. Before you buy, check for good functional design. The key words are safe, sturdy, efficient, easy to work, easy to fix. Look for these features when you buy a house, a motor home, a car, shoes, a toothbrush, or anything else. As a consumer, you speak with your dollars—and that's the language the designers ultimately listen to. When you run into something particularly outrageous, write the manufacturer. Write a consumer group. Write a government consumer agency. Keep the pressure on.

Meanwhile, here are a few hints to help you with the world as it now is.

Home Treatment

The car-door push-button device is truly a beast—you have to push with the thumb and pull with the hand at the same time, and the thumb action is against a hard spring. Some-

times you will be able to push the button with your palm. If not, try both thumbs at once. Or, you can have a handyman make an aluminum gripper that hooks on the door handle and lets you lever the push button in. New car door handles are easier than those of older cars; if you have trouble with the catch, a T-shaped piece of wood will let you pry it up.

A handle with pointed bars, as some shower handles, can also be worked with a lever—a bamboo or aluminum tube works well. When you buy new fixtures, however, get ones with a single lever that controls both water force and temperature. Remember the lever, because it is the answer to a lot of frustrating problems.

When you grip, learn to use the palm. If you press on a handle, you get a surprising amount of friction. By then rotating the whole hand, you can turn the handle without actually gripping it. You can use a little grip too, but let the friction of the hand do most of the work.

Keys can be built up with an added wooden handle to make them easier to turn. But don't forget the graphite. With a little lock oil or graphite in the lock, the whole job becomes much easier.

What to Expect from the Health Professional

The occupational therapist can give you additional adaptive suggestions and is a good person to ask about where to obtain some of the materials you need. Again, the *Self-Help Manual* of the Arthritis Foundation is another useful aid to locating ideas and resources.

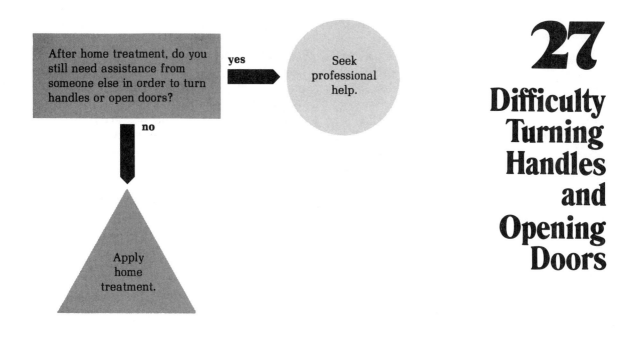

After home treatment, do you still need assistance from someone else in order to turn handles or open doors?

yes → Seek professional help.

no ↓

Apply home treatment.

27
Difficulty Turning Handles and Opening Doors

28

Problems Opening Jars

Some people think that apple-sauce jars are the worst. Others give the award to catsup bottles. Then there are the can openers, and the plastic or cellophane that won't tear. These are problems for everyone. Domestic battles rage over the opening of a difficult jar on a difficult day. And if your grip strength is decreased because of arthritis, you may need some tricks to help you out (with the jars, not the domestic battles).

Don't minimize this problem because it seems so ordinary and so unimportant. Frustration at a trivial task is more marked than with a larger one. Your feeling of helplessness before a stubborn jar is not good for you. So learn the tricks.

Home Treatment

Mount a wedge-shaped gripper on the kitchen wall; this allows you to turn the jar easily with two hands while the lid is securely held. Break the suction on vacuum lids, such as apple sauce, with a "lid lifter" available in houseware departments everywhere. Use a fork handle as a lever to pull up ring-top openers.

With boxes, lie the box on its side and cut the top off with a knife. Use scissors for sealed plastic or cellophane.

Get an electric can opener. The ones that have a power stroke to pierce the can will save you additional effort. If you use a hand can opener, make sure that the keys are large and easy to grip.

Practice opening jars with your palm. The friction between lid and palm enables you to get more force than you can with just the grip. You can use a little grip to assist the palm friction. This simple but unfamiliar action can make opening jars a lot easier.

What to Expect from the Health Professional

The occupational therapist can suggest some additional tricks and is a good person to ask for places to obtain items. Everything you need to conquer this particular problem is probably available at a nearby store, so the health professional will not be of as much assistance. You have to learn to look for items with care, anticipating how well they will work with your particular disability.

After home treatment, do you still need assistance from someone else in order to open moderately difficult cans or jars?

yes → Seek professional help.

no

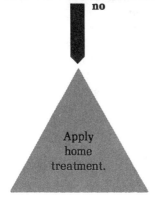

Apply home treatment.

28
Problems Opening Jars

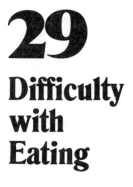

29

Difficulty with Eating

This is a most fundamental frustration. Eating is a complicated task that involves mental activity, physical abilities, and body reflexes to carry the food to and through the stomach. Interruption of the sequence at any point can cause a problem. The problem for the person with arthritis may involve difficulty in cutting the food, in getting the food to the mouth, in chewing, or in swallowing. These problems affect only a very few patients with arthritis, but they are serious ones. Eating is a social occasion as well as a biological necessity, and eating gracefully without self-consciousness is a social skill we take for granted.

Home Treatment

The suggestions here are just to get you started. As with other daily activities, your own solutions will require a bit of personal input and ingenuity.

There are several ways to make it easier to cut your food. Attractive utensils are available with big handles that enable you to get a better grip. If the plate is placed on a damp sponge cloth or a thin disk of rubber, it will not slip while you are cutting. This may give you an extra hand for the knife as well as a feeling of greater security. Don't forget that a sharp knife will cut more easily than a dull one. Or that foods can be selected which are equally good in taste but easier to cut. High-friction plastic placed between the plate and the table will keep the plate steady while you cut. These measures can help in stirring or opening as well as in cutting. Check with your occupational therapist for sources near you.

In getting food to the mouth, built-up utensil handles are again useful. T-handled cups make for an easier grip, as does a terry-cloth coaster around a glass. Long-handled utensils are needed by some, while angled utensils are easier for others. A swivel spoon can be used by patients unable to twist their wrist to bring liquid to the mouth. Straws are sometimes an easy way to drink, and an ordinary pencil clip can help you attach the straw to the side of the glass to make it even simpler.

Chewing problems can arise from arthritis of the jaw joints or from problems with the teeth or the chewing muscles. Good dental care is essential. Selection of food that can be easily chewed is one way to avoid the problem.

Swallowing can be affected in several ways. In myositis, the upper swallowing muscles may not work. In scleroderma, the muscles in the lower gullet may not pass a smooth swallowing wave. Medicines given for arthritis may irritate the stomach and not let food leave the stomach efficiently. Chew carefully and slowly and swallow carefully. If the problem seems to be low in the gullet, and antacid may be helpful. Take small, frequent meals, use softer-textured foods, take liquids with meals, and eat and chew slowly. Try not eating for the two or three hours before bedtime if you have pain behind the breastbone when you eat. Having pain when you eat is an indication that you should see the doctor, as is any weight loss due to difficulty eating.

What to Expect from the Health Professional

The occupational therapist is knowledgable about adaptive aids and where to get them. The social worker may be needed in severe cases to locate public resources. The doctor is necessary if chewing or swallowing problems are causing major difficulty. X-rays of the jaw and the temporomandibular joint may be taken. An upper-GI series is an X-ray of the esophagus, stomach, and duodenum, and it may help identify a problem in these areas.

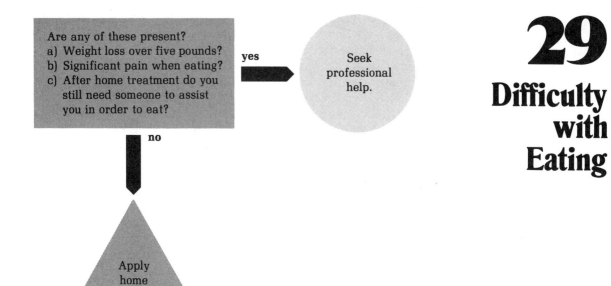

Are any of these present?
a) Weight loss over five pounds?
b) Significant pain when eating?
c) After home treatment do you still need someone to assist you in order to eat?

yes

Seek professional help.

no

Apply home treatment.

29
Difficulty with Eating

30
Problems with Stairs

In some living environments, there are no stairs. This is true of the single-level house or homes equipped with elevators. In other situations, the ability to climb stairs is essential to independent life. Stairs sometimes must be used several times a day; even the bathroom, if upstairs, can require this activity.

Problems with the knees, with the hips, or with the quadriceps muscles in the thigh are usually responsible for difficulty with stairs. Thus, loss of the ability to climb stairs is a signal for increased attention to the arthritis problem; a minor problem has just become major.

Home Treatment

Often, your first approach should be to check the treatment program for your arthritis. Are you taking the medication regularly? Does your doctor have further suggestions? Are you working on your quadriceps-strengthening exercises? Might a steroid injection of an inflamed knee be of benefit? Is this the signal to consider seriously a surgical procedure on the bad hip or knee?

Sometimes you can rearrange your environment quite a bit. Should you move? An apartment with an elevator? A ranch-style house with a single level? Should you remodel? A downstairs bedroom and bath? A ramp in the garden, gently graded? Such changes can sometimes render the stairs unnecessary.

Can you improve your stairs? Be sure you have a rail or bannister on each side, so that you can both steady yourself and push a bit with your arms. Sometimes installation of a center rail will help you by allowing you to use both hands at once. The split-riser trick also helps some people. If your problem is that the steps are just too high, you can have a carpenter install split risers, so that half of each step is raised half a step, alternating left and right. Then you can climb the stairs, moving back and forth, without ever having to go up a full step at a time.

The rule for climbing stairs: one at a time, with both feet on the same stair before trying the next one. Go up with the best leg first; go down with the best leg first. Use the same technique for curbs.

Another possibility is installation of a home elevator or lift that goes up on a bannister. These are fairly expensive and are thus out of reach for all but a few. If you are considering one of these, you should think through the option of moving or remodeling again.

What to Expect from the Health Professional

The occupational therapist may have some additional suggestions for you and will know where to obtain materials and help. The social worker may be able to help with sources of financing. Remember that changes in your living arrangements, like stairs, necessitated by your arthritis are tax deductible. Thus, the actual cost will be a little less than you first expect.

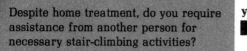
Despite home treatment, do you require assistance from another person for necessary stair-climbing activities?

yes

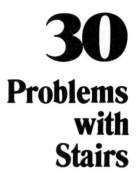
Seek professional help.

30
Problems with Stairs

no

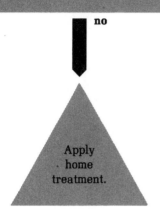
Apply home treatment.

31
Difficulty Walking

Walking is central to almost every other activity. The ability to walk must be preserved. If walking is impaired, the muscles become weak, the bones lose calcium, friends are more distant, and the easiest tasks become formidable. This cycle can further reduce your health and increase your dependency on others.

So, if you are having trouble walking and you can't take care of the problem yourself, have a long talk with your doctor. Usually, something can be done. The longer that you have been unable to walk, the more difficult the solution.

With arthritis, fatigue can cause a decrease in your desire to walk; this must be combatted. Or, problems with the ball of the foot, the ankles, the knees, the hips, or the walking muscles can be responsible for the difficulty. It is partly a medical problem and partly a social one.

Home Treatment

Be sure that the treatment for your arthritis is right. Are you taking your medication regularly? Do you need a change in medication? Could this be a side effect of a medication? Is your exercise program progressing smoothly? Is a single joint causing the trouble? Could this joint be injected? Do you perhaps have a joint infection? Is this the time to consider surgery for that knee or hip? These and similar questions will help you decide on a strategy to get walking again.

A cane is the simplest aid to walking. It is usually held in the hand opposite an affected hip and on the most comfortable side for a bad knee. The usual C-handled cane is not really designed to be held easily, so you might prefer one with a functional grip handle. Some handles may need to be built up with tape to allow a good grip.

Crutches give somewhat more support but are more cumbersome. When using crutches, your weight should not be on your armpits but on your arms. You may have to pad the grip or fit a knob to the crutch to get a good grip. The armpit is laced with fragile nerves and blood vessels and pressure there for very long can cause damage. If your grip is not too good, forearm platform crutches help you take the weight on the forearm. Bags can be attached to the crutch to allow small items to be carried—you just don't have enough hands for a purse or a package otherwise.

Walkers give stable support but are difficult to use for long distances. They are most useful about the house and while you're getting back on your feet after a flare-up or operation.

Don't forget the importance of correct footwear. If foot pain is limiting your walking, you will want to refer to some of the hints given in problem 7 or problem 8.

Then there are gliders and wheelchairs. These are a subject in themselves. Good information is available in the *Self-Help Manual* of the Arthritis Foundation or from your physical therapist or occupational therapist. The goal, of course, is to keep you out of a wheelchair; each of the measures mentioned above helps you strengthen your body.

What to Expect from the Health Professional

The physical therapist will help you get started with appliances for walking assistance and will instruct you in exercises to strengthen your legs. The occupational therapist can help with additional adaptive devices. Social workers may assist in mobilizing community resources to help you. Your doctor will want to take a very serious look at your treatment program to ensure that all of the right things are being done.

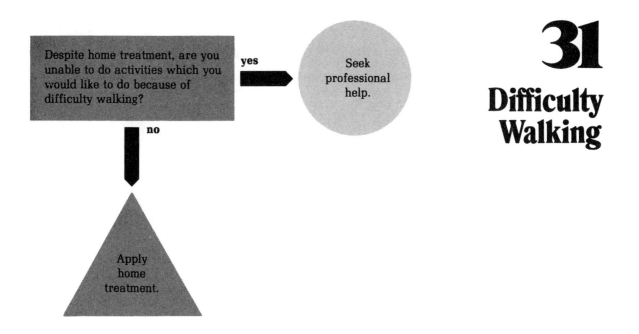

31

Difficulty Walking

14
Sexual Problems

Problems with sexual relationships occur much more often than would be suspected from the frequency of their discussion. Surprisingly, the patient is often not consciously aware of a sexual problem. Or, the patient may be embarrassed to bring the subject up, especially an older patient who feels that sexual problems are not supposed to be an issue at certain ages. The doctor seldom asks specifically about sexual problems. Books either omit the subject or include a glib discussion about finding more comfortable sexual positions.

There is no single solution to these complex problems. There are as many different kinds of sexual needs and preferences as there are personalities. Trying to match some arbitrary definition of normal is exactly what you do not want to do. Instead, you should seek what is comfortable for you and your partner. Your own decisions will be determined by your background, your preferences before you had arthritis, the availability of a partner, and the needs and preferences of that partner. Problems can be discussed under the three categories of frustration, manipulation, and guilt.

FRUSTRATION

This is the problem that comes first to mind, and the one that may be most easily managed. Basically, the frustrated person wants and needs sexual release, but cannot obtain it with sufficient frequency. The motive is there—the problem is one of opportunity and means. Perhaps the patient's self-image, diminished by arthritis, impedes the initiation of a sexual encounter. Perhaps there is no partner. Perhaps the process of sexual rela-

231

tions is painful. Perhaps disability limits performance. Perhaps a drug taken for the arthritis is decreasing sexual ability.

Self-image is critically important to sexual function. In this book, we've repeatedly stressed the dangers of perceiving yourself as a "victim" or an "invalid." You need confidence to face the challenges imposed by your arthritis. Sexual function can mirror your general opinion of yourself. The emotional aspects of sex are more important than the physical. Loneliness, depression, and isolation are more damaging than sexual abstinence. Sexual relationships can be a way of enhancing your self-image and the general level of your personal satisfactions.

From this viewpoint, you can avoid sexual failure even though technical difficulties with sexual performance persist. You can be sexually attractive. Attractiveness is related to caring, to careful listening, to respect for your partner. Dress attractively. Control your body weight. Groom carefully. The sexual solutions may well follow renewed respect for yourself.

The missing partner is a frequent and often overlooked problem. Sexual frequency in older individuals is strongly related to the availability of a sexual partner. Since women live considerably longer, on the average, than do men, the problem is usually that of a widow, and is aggravated if the person is living alone with few social contacts. Sometimes sex is not a problem at all in this setting; if it is not, do not make it one. There is no rule that says there is no life after sex. If you do have a problem, masturbation is a possible answer. Medically, this is an excellent means of physical release, but the guilt experienced by some people prevents it from being a perfect solution. Seeking a partner is a neglected solution that can be thoroughly satisfactory at any age. The thrill of the September courtship is often as intense as that of young lovers, and many problems associated with arthritis are greatly helped by the presence of a partner.

If sexual relationships are painful, there are a number of possible steps you can take. Keep in mind that prolonged foreplay increases vaginal lubrication and eases penetration, decreasing effort and pain. A vaginal lubricant, such as KY Jelly, may be used. Rheumatoid arthritis, in particular, often has vaginal dryness as one of its complications, so don't interpret lack of lubrication as sexual dysfunction. Better control of the arthritis will help, so discuss medications with your doctor. Anti-inflammatory medicine, taken two hours before intercourse, can help. Avoid painkillers, since they often depress desire and sexual function. Urinate prior to intercourse. Take a warm bath if it helps you relax and loosen up. Use music to partially distract you from minor discomfort. Get comfortable in anticipation.

Position during intercourse can be varied, by trial and error, to find the most satisfactory. There is no single most satisfactory position. The standard advice is for the partner with arthritis to assume the more passive, usually underneath, role—but this does *not* consistently work. Sometimes one side or the other, male-inferior, male-superior, or posterior-entry positions work better. Some patients get a lot of benefit from using such simple devices as knee pads to protect sore knees or a pillow beneath the buttocks.

Manual stimulation and oral stimulation can be less strenuous aspects of the love act.

Consider the best time of day to have sexual relations, particularly if you are bothered by fatigue in the afternoon or stiffness in the morning. For some, the middle of the day is most satisfactory. The more experimentation you feel comfortable with, the greater your chances of hitting the right combination. But don't force your emotional comfort; don't attempt sexual maneuvers that make you feel emotionally uncomfortable.

Disability can absolutely limit sexual activity, but this is extremely rare. Contractures of both hips in a female is the most frequent of such problems and may well be a signal for consideration of a surgical approach.

Drugs are a frequently overlooked cause of sexual dysfunction. Alcohol, painkillers, sedatives, and tranquilizers all depress desire and ability, although in small doses each may act to facilitate relaxation. Drugs given to control a problem with the blood pressure pose a more direct problem; Aldomet and Ismelin, for example, very frequently impair male sexual function. Suspect almost any drug and talk with your doctor about it. If a drug is causing impotence, then the solution is simple. You just stop the drug or substitute a different drug.

MANIPULATION

This problem is major, frequent, and seldom recognized either by the manipulating partner or the one being manipulated. Here, one partner is using arthritis to avoid sexual encounters or to make the other feel badly about the imposition. This problem is rooted in the relationship, not in the sex itself. Obesity has recently been identified as being, in some individuals, a mechanism to decrease sexual attractiveness and to thus avoid stresses related to sexual encounters. Arthritis can, on occasion, be used in the same way. The sexual dysfunction in such cases will be out of proportion to the actual physical problem. This mechanism is similar to the classic "I've got a headache" technique for postponement of sexual activity. This is a big problem: the secondary gain (avoidance of sex) the patient gets from being disabled leads to therapeutic frustration—the patient doesn't really want to be well.

The same passive manipulation technique can be used in reverse by the nonarthritic partner. Here, sexual difficulties are interpreted as deliberate aggravation, even though the disability and problems are real. The partner without arthritis is trying to increase guilt and to decrease the self-image of the partner with arthritis—sort of a revenge tactic.

These problems are very hard to recognize and often harder to solve. The answer is, of course, for both partners to open up direct channels of communication and to negotiate, as adults, for the best solution: "It's not really the arthritis so much; I just really would like to have sex less often." "I get frustrated because of your arthritis, and I guess I've been pushing you on sex to try and get rid of my anger." If such communication can develop, a negotiated solution is usually possible. The techniques of the previous section may be helpful. If the needs of the partners remain far apart, the entire relationship needs careful assessment. Marriage counselors or sexual counseling can help. But these problems usually were present before the arthritis, and such deep-rooted habit patterns are extremely difficult to change.

GUILT

The best sex relationships are free of guilt. This means greatly different things to different people; there can be no rigid rules. Most recent discussions of sex have been condemnations of old sexual taboos; sensual experiences previously considered deviant are now vigorously encouraged. This has generated a sort of reverse guilt in some. Now one can be guilty for *not* doing, while previously one was made to feel guilty for doing.

The sexual styles of different generations vary like shirt collars or skirt lengths. There is no single right answer, and the general rules fall before the particular instance. Some people feel awkward or undignified with certain sexual positions. Some find oral sex distasteful or experience prolonged guilt after masturbation. What is biologically equivalent may not be emotionally equivalent. Guilt over some sexual practice, guilt over nonperformance, guilt over infrequency, guilt over abstinence—all of these are detrimental. The practices with which you and your partner are most comfortable are the right ones. There is no norm. It is your sex life.

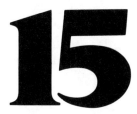

Problems with Employment

Winston Churchill used to follow a political and military strategy of "keeping all options open." This is the basic employment strategy for a person with significant arthritis.

PROBLEMS AND REALITIES

Let's look at some typical problems. A woman patient with recent onset of rheumatoid arthritis experiences fatigue, depression, and a problem with adjustment. Treatment has not yet been very helpful. She begins to work more slowly, misses some time, and her employer notes that her value to the company is decreasing. Her perception of failure on the job results in more depression and the cycle continues until she either quits or gets fired.

A patient with Reiter's syndrome is unable to carry out work duties because of painful feet and ankles. Or, advanced osteoarthritis of the knees causes a patient sufficient pain and disability to contemplate surgery—and lost time. Or, a patient with inflamed finger joints from rheumatoid arthritis is advised not to work at an occupation that requires heavy use of the hands.

There are many such scenarios. Arthritis, defined broadly, causes more disability and more time lost than any other set of human conditions.

Now let's look at the realities. That new rheumatoid arthritis patient will adjust to the problem and the disease will be controlled by medication. The Reiter's syndrome will subside as the particular flare-up ends. The contemplated knee surgery will restore function and decrease pain for the immobile patient with osteoarthritis. The inflamed finger joints, over months, will become much better, and that patient will accept a better-paying job in the accounting department. Each of these patients will become employable again and each will do a good job.

Work is a very positive thing. It promotes independence, self-fulfillment and problem-solving skills. It provides money, which decreases one set of worries. It encourages active social interaction with other people. We like our patients to go on working despite their arthritis and to return to work if they have to stop temporarily. The pain message and your common sense will tell you what you can do.

THE BAD NEWS AND THE GOOD NEWS

Unfortunately, there is a negative side to the employment question, and it reflects poorly on our society. The patient with arthritis has been neglected by the politician and by the social planner. Sick leave, medical insurance, unemployment programs, and disability awards are not designed for the intermediate term of six to twelve months, and they often discriminate against musculoskeletal disability.

Sometimes if you return to work from disability status you lose the right to go back on it if things don't work out. What a crazy system! Sometimes an employer will discriminate, in spite of Fair Employment Practices Acts, against patients with arthritis, fearing that their productivity will be lower and their sick time more frequent.

Political lobbies for the disabled have concentrated on the paraplegic patient and the patient with spinal-cord injuries instead of the much more common problem of arthritis. Definitions of "physically handicapped" are often narrow, excluding patients with arthritis. The situation is lamentably inflexible. Our view is that disability arrangements are rarely required for the arthritis patient, but when they are needed, it is gross injustice for them to be difficult to obtain. Your support of the Arthritis Foundation, nationally and locally, can help improve this situation.

Now the better news. Social solutions can be found. Be persistent with public officials and insurance companies. It helps if you have a doctor or social worker who knows the local situation well. Several letters from the doctor may be needed. Highly placed officials of some insurance plans have told me that first claims for payment are automatically rejected by the computer, but that follow-up requests are then evaluated on their merits. So be persistent.

HOW TO HELP YOURSELF

Then there is your part. As always, you play the biggest role in solving your problems. The hints in the previous problem discussions will help. Your expectations must be both positive and realistic. And you must be determined.

Figure out your prognosis. Check the questionnaire in Appendix A to find out how bad your arthritis is; pay particular attention to your "disability index" score. Read the general prognosis for your kind of arthritis in Part I. And remember that after a year or so of arthritis you can predict the future pretty well by analyzing the past; you are unlikely to get any new problems after that period.

Is your present job right for you? Retraining or job transfer is best accomplished if there isn't any rush and if you are employed at the time of inquiry. Wait for the right opening and transfer into it. If you anticipate slowly increasing difficulty with a particular activity, make plans to avoid that activity.

The patient with significant arthritis usually has major advantages over persons with other handicaps. Most importantly, the brain works fine. So do the heart and the lungs. The person beneath the outward infirmity is well equipped to adjust to problems with pain or mobility.

The adjustment is not easy and it would be nice if the System were more hassle-free, but employment problems can be solved. Productive life despite arthritis is the goal, and it can be achieved.

PART

IV

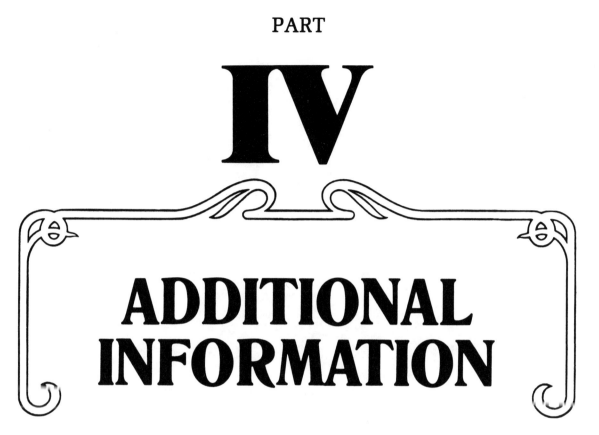

ADDITIONAL
INFORMATION

A

Rate Your Arthritis

This Arthritis Status Test is used by arthritis centers to evaluate the status of their patients. You can score your own arthritis and you can follow your own progress over time. For reference, compare your scores with those of patients at the Stanford Arthritis Center.

THE ARTHRITIS STATUS TEST

Mark lightly with a pencil (you will want to use this test again) the one response that best describes your abilities as they usually are now.

	Without difficulty	*With difficulty*	*With help from another*	*Unable to do at all*
Daily Function				
1. Dressing: Can you get your clothes, dress yourself, shampoo your hair . . .	0	1	2	3
2. Standing up: Are you able to stand up from a straight chair without using your arms to push off . . .	0	1	2	3

	Without difficulty	With difficulty	With help from another	Unable to do at all
3. Eating: Can you cut your meat and lift a cup to your mouth . . .	0	1	2	3
4. Walking: Can you walk outdoors on flat ground . . .	0	1	2	3
5. Hygiene: Can you wash and dry your entire body, turn faucets, and get on and off the toilet . . .	0	1	2	3
6. Reach: Can you reach up to and get down a seven-pound object that is above your head . . .	0	1	2	3
7. Grip: Can you open push-button car doors and jars that have been previously opened . . .	0	1	2	3
8. Activity: Can you drive a car or run errands and shop . . .	0	1	2	3

	Without difficulty	Somewhat painful or no sexual partner	Very painful	Impossible because of arthritis
9. Sex: Are you able to have sexual relations . . .	0	1	2	3

Pain and Discomfort

	None	Mild	Moderate	Severe
1. Severity: How would you describe the pain from your arthritis over the past week?	0	1	2	3

2. Trend: How has the severity of the pain changed over the past week?

No pain	Better	The same	Worse
0	1	2	3

That's the test. Now, put the numbers (0, 1, 2, 3) corresponding to your answers in the appropriate spaces of the first column of the Arthritis Rating Sheet that follows. The other columns are for repeating the test in the future; we recommend every six months. You must have answered all of the questions to have a valid score.

THE ARTHRITIS RATING SHEET

Date taken _____ _____ _____ _____ _____ _____

Daily Function

1. Dressing _____ _____ _____ _____ _____ _____

2. Standing up _____ _____ _____ _____ _____ _____

3. Eating _____ _____ _____ _____ _____ _____

4. Walking _____ _____ _____ _____ _____ _____

5. Hygiene _____ _____ _____ _____

6. Reach _____ _____ _____ _____ _____ _____

7. Grip _____ _____ _____ _____ _____ _____

8. Activity _____ _____ _____ _____ _____ _____

9. Sex _____ _____ _____ _____ _____ _____

Function points (Add 1 through 9) _____ _____ _____ _____ _____ _____

Pain and Discomfort

1. Severity _____ _____ _____ _____ _____ _____

2. Trend _____ _____ _____ _____ _____ _____

Pain points (Add 1 and 2) _____ _____ _____ _____ _____ _____

HOW TO INTERPRET YOUR SCORE

This status test has been used with over 500 patients with rheumatoid arthritis evaluated by the Stanford Arthritis Center. These persons have had arthritis for an average of five to ten years, and have worse arthritis than the typical patient. You can compare your score with the figures below, which show the percentage of patients with different numbers of points.

Function points

Points	Rating	Percent of RA patients
0–4	Normal	36 percent
5–13	Adequate	47 percent
14–22	Impaired	16 percent
23–27	Disabled	1 percent

Pain points

Points	Rating	Percent of RA patients
0	None	2 percent
1–2	Mild	8 percent
3–4	Moderate	64 percent
5–6	Severe	26 percent

Repeat your scoring each six months and date and record the results. You will be able to measure your improvement. If your scores are getting worse, it may be time to talk with your doctor about changing your treatment program.

B

Additional Resources

A READING LIST

The following materials provide additional discussions of the topics in this book. I believe them to be basically sound and of potential value for the patient with arthritis.

Recommended Books about Arthritis and Rheumatism

Bland, John H., M.D. *Arthritis Medical Treatment and Home Care.* London: Collier Macmillan, 1960.

Blau, Sheldon, M.D., and Dodi Schultz. *Arthritis.* Garden City, N.Y.: Doubleday, 1973.

Calabro, John J., M.D., and John Wykert. *The Truth about Arthritis Care.* New York: McKay, 1971.

Friedmann, Lawrence W., M.D. *Freedom from Backaches.* New York: Simon and Schuster, 1973.

Healey, Louis A., M.D., Kenneth Wilske, M.D., and Bob Hansen. *Beyond the Copper Bracelet.* 2d ed. Bowie, Maryland: The Charles Press, 1977.

Jayson, Malcolm V., M.D., and Alan St. J. Dixon, M.D. *Understanding Arthritis and Rheumatism.* New York: Dell, 1974.

Johnson, G. Timothy, M.D. *Coping with Arthritis.* New York: Newspaperbooks, 1977.

Kraus, Hans, M.D. *The Cause, Prevention, and Treatment of Backache, Stress, and Tension.* New York: Simon and Schuster, 1965.

Not Recommended

I believe these books to be oversimplified or misleading, sometimes dangerously so. They are given by title only.

There Is a Cure for Arthritis

Arthritis Can Be Cured

A Doctor's Proven New Home Cure for Arthritis

The Arthritic's Cookbook

New Hope for the Arthritic

Arthritis and Folk Medicine

Your Aching Back and What You Can Do About It

Arthritis, Nutrition, and Natural Therapy

Arthritis and Common Sense

Pamphlets Available from the Arthritis Foundation

Excellent pamphlets are available through your local chapter office of the Arthritis Foundation or from the national Arthritis Foundation office. Usually there is no charge for single copies; there is often a nominal charge for multiple copies to cover printing costs. Titles change; you should consult your local chapter for presently available materials. Here are a few good ones.

Arthritis: The Basic Facts. 28 pages.

Self-Help Manual for Arthritis Patients. ($1.25) 124 pages. Excellent.

Must be ordered by health professional

Primer on the Rheumatic Diseases ($1.00)

THE ARTHRITIS FOUNDATION

The "AF" is a truly marvelous institution. It sponsors programs in public education and professional education, supports young doctors establishing research careers in arthritis, and provides direct support for research activities. The meetings of the American Rheumatism Association (ARA), a section of the Arthritis Foundation, provide the principal forum for discussion of new scientific knowledge about arthritis. The AF leads the fight for increased government programs of research and service.

The Arthritis Foundation consists of a national office and local chapters around the country. You will usually want to contact the local chapter, which can advise you of doctors and clinics in your area, provide instructional materials, and occasionally may be able to help with financial problems. The pamphlets listed above should be available from your local chapter. There may be a schedule of activities you might wish to attend. Or you might want to volunteer your efforts in support of the chapter.

National Office

The Arthritis Foundation
3400 Peachtree Road, N.E.—Room 1101
Atlanta, Georgia 30326
Telephone: (404) 266-0795

Arthritis foundation chapters

Alabama

Alabama Chapter
13 Office Park Circle—Room 14
Birmingham, Alabama 35223
205-870-4700

South Alabama Chapter
304 Little Flower Avenue
Mobile, Alabama 36606
205-471-1725

Arizona

Central Arizona Chapter
100 West Osborn—Suite D
Phoenix, Arizona 85013
602-264-7679

Southern Arizona Chapter
3833 East Second Street
Tucson, Arizona 85716
602-326-2811

Arkansas

Arkansas Chapter
6213 Lee Avenue
Little Rock, Arkansas 72205
501-664-7242

California

Northeastern California Chapter
3560 "J" Street
Sacramento, California 95816
916-452-5343

Northern California Chapter
399 Buena Vista Avenue East

San Francisco, California 94117
415-621-3976

San Diego Area Chapter
3719 Fourth Avenue
San Diego, California 92103
714-291-0430

Southern California Chapter
4311 Wilshire Boulevard
Los Angeles, California 90010
213-938-6111

Colorado

Rocky Mountain Chapter
70 W. Sixth Avenue—Room 209
Denver, Colorado 80204
303-623-5191

Connecticut

Connecticut Chapter
929 Silas Deane Highway
Wethersfield, Connecticut 06109
203-563-1177

Delaware

Delaware Chapter
234 Philadelphia Pike—Suite 3
Wilmington, Delaware 19809
302-764-8254

District of Columbia

Arthritis and Rheumatism Assoc.
of Metropolitan Washington
2424 Pennsylvania Ave. N.W. #105
Washington, D.C. 20037
202-331-7395

Florida

Florida Chapter
3205 Manatee Ave. West
Bradenton, Florida 33505
813-748-1300

Georgia

Georgia Chapter
2799 Delk Road, S.E.
Marietta, Georgia 30067
404-952-4254

Hawaii

Hawaii Chapter
200 North Vineyard—Suite 505
Honolulu, Hawaii 96817
808-531-1920

Idaho

Idaho Chapter
6003 Overland Road
Boise, Idaho 83705
208-376-5831

Illinois

Central Illinois Chapter
Allied Agencies Center
320 East Armstrong Ave.—Rm. 102
Peoria, Illinois 61603
309-672-6337

Illinois Chapter
79 W. Monroe—Suite 1105
Chicago, Illinois 60603
312-782-1367

Indiana

Indiana Chapter
1010 East 86th Street
Indianapolis, Indiana 46240
317-844-3341

Iowa

Iowa Chapter
215 Keo Way—Suite 314
Des Moines, Iowa 50309
515-243-6259

Kansas

Kansas Chapter
1602 East Waterman
Wichita, Kansas 67211
316-263-0116

Kentucky

Kentucky Chapter
1381 Bardstown Road
Louisville, Kentucky 40204
502-459-6460

Louisiana

Louisiana Chapter
1215 Dublin Street
New Orleans, Louisiana 70118
504-861-4673

Maine

Maine Chapter
141 Front Street
Bath, Maine 04530
207-442-8109

Maryland

Maryland Chapter
12 West 25th Street
Baltimore, Maryland 21218
301-366-0923

Massachusetts

Massachusetts Chapter
38 Chauncy Street—Room 611
Boston, Massachusetts 02111
617-542-6535

Michigan

Michigan Chapter
23400 Michigan Ave.—Suite 605
Dearborn, Michigan 48124
313-561-9096

Minnesota

Minnesota Chapter
122 West Franklin—Suite 440
Minneapolis, Minnesota 55404
612-874-1201

Mississippi

Mississippi Chapter
5360 I-55 North, Room 303
Jackson, Mississippi 39211
601-956-3371

Missouri

Eastern Missouri Chapter
P.O. Box 1144
St. Louis, Missouri 63188
314-421-3550

Kansas City Chapter
2727 Main Street
Kansas City, Missouri 64108
816-221-5383

Montana

Midland Montana Chapter
1201 Avenue C
Billings, Montana 59102
406-259-4451

North Montana Chapter
P.O. Box 2383
Great Falls, Montana 59403
406-453-6511

Western Montana Chapter
1575 West Sussex Street
Missoula, Montana 59801
406-549-0964

Nebraska

Nebraska Chapter
120 North 69th Street—Room 202
Omaha, Nebraska 68132
402-588-2400

New Hampshire

New Hampshire Chapter
P.O. Box 369
Concord, New Hampshire 03301
603-224-9322

New Jersey

New Jersey Chapter
26 Prospect Street

Westfield, New Jersey 07090
201-233-7151

New Mexico

New Mexico Chapter
5112 Grand Avenue, N. E.
Albuquerque, New Mexico 87108
505-265-1545

New York

Central New York Chapter
700 E. Water Street—Room 108
Syracuse, New York 13210
315-422-8174

Monroe County Chapter
973 East Avenue
Rochester, New York 14607
716-271-3540

New York Chapter
221 Park Avenue South
New York, New York 10003
212-677-5790

Northeastern New York Chapter
11 North Pearl Street—Room 707
Albany, New York 12207
518-434-4122

Western New York Chapter
742 Delaware Avenue
Buffalo, New York 14209
716-887-2639

North Carolina

North Carolina Chapter
P.O. Box 2505
Durham, North Carolina 27705
919-477-0286

North Dakota

Dakota Chapter
410 N. Broadway
Fargo, North Dakota 58102
701-232-6282

Ohio

Akron Area Chapter
326 Locust Street

Akron, Ohio 44302
216-253-1171

Central Ohio Chapter
2501 N. Star Road
Columbus, Ohio 43221
614-488-0777

Northeastern Ohio Chapter
2239 East 55th Street
Cleveland, Ohio 44103
216-361-5000

Northwestern Ohio Chapter
3817 Monroe Street
Toledo, Ohio 43606
419-473-3349

Southwestern Ohio Chapter
2400 Reading Road
Cincinnati, Ohio 45202
513-721-1027

Oklahoma

Eastern Oklahoma Chapter
3365 E. Skelly Drive
Tulsa, Oklahoma 74135
918-749-1394

Oklahoma Chapter
3313 Classen Boulevard—Suite 101
Oklahoma City, Oklahoma 73118
405-521-0066

Oregon

Oregon Chapter
P.O. Box 42067
Portland, Oregon 97242
503-234-0404

Pennsylvania

Central Pennsylvania Chapter
P.O. Box 534
Harrisburg, Pennsylvania 17108
717-234-2661

Eastern Pennsylvania Chapter
311 So. Juniper Street—Suite 1008
Philadelphia, Pennsylvania 19107
215-735-5272

Western Pennsylvania Chapter
6115 Jenkins Arcade
Pittsburgh, Pennsylvania 15222
412-566-1645/6

Rhode Island

Rhode Island Chapter
49 Weybosset Street
Providence, Rhode Island 02903
401-421-4410

South Carolina

South Carolina Chapter
3008 Millwood Avenue
Columbia, South Carolina 29205
803-254-6702

South Dakota (see *North Dakota*)

Tennessee

Middle-East Tennessee Chapter
1719 West End Building
Nashville, Tennessee 37203
615-329-3431

West Tennessee Chapter
2600 Poplar Avenue—Suite 200
Memphis, Tennessee 38112
901-452-4482

Texas

North Texas Chapter
5415 Maple Avenue—Suite 416
Dallas, Texas 75235
214-638-7474

Northwest Texas Chapter
3145 McCart Street
Fort Worth, Texas 76110
817-926-7733

South Central Texas Chapter
8000 Vantage Drive—Room 108
San Antonio, Texas 78230
512-349-0171

Texas Gulf Coast Chapter
4848 Guiton #116
Houston, Texas 77027
713-626-2680

West Texas Chapter
3701 North Big Spring
Midland, Texas 79701
915-684-5864

Utah

Utah Chapter
Graystone Plaza, #4
1174 E. 2700 South
Salt Lake City, Utah 84106
801-466-9389

Vermont

Vermont Chapter
215 College Street
Burlington, Vermont 05401
802-864-4988

Virginia

Virginia Chapter
P.O. Box 5069
Richmond, Virginia 23220
804-353-4471

Washington

Western Washington Chapter
Dexter Horton Building, Room 522
710 2nd Avenue
Seattle, Washington 98104
206-622-2481

West Virginia

West Virginia Chapter
440 Fourth Avenue
South Charleston, W. Va. 25303
304-744-3042

Wisconsin

Wisconsin Chapter
611 E. Wells Street
Milwaukee, Wisconsin 53202
414-276-0490

Wyoming (see *Colorado*)

HOW YOU CAN HELP

You can provide valuable assistance to the fight against arthritis. Learn about the issues from the Arthritis Foundation and support increased national committment to more research and better care. Write your senator and congressman; ask for increased appropriations under the National Arthritis Act.

Support arthritis research and care programs directly. You can contribute at any of the three levels listed below. Contributions are tax deductible. Bequests are extremely helpful to the arthritis battle and you can ask about arrangements for a "living will."

The Arthritis Foundation (national office). Mail letters and checks to the address given in the previous section.

The Arthritis Foundation (your local chapter). Mail letters and checks to the address of your local chapter as listed above under the heading of your state.

University research programs in arthritis. Contact the university of your choice for information about their research programs and instructions for contributions. Contributions may be designated for training of young physicians or for research into a particular disease.

Our Stanford program may be supported by contributions to the following addresses. If a bequest or memorial, send checks to:

■ Arthritis Memorial Research Fund—Stanford University
Department of Medicine, S102B
Stanford University School of Medicine
Stanford, California 94305

If a gift, send checks to:

■ Research Gift Fund, Dr. J. F. Fries—Stanford University
Department of Medicine, S102B
Stanford University School of Medicine
Stanford, California 94305

Index

255

Synovectomy, 131
Synovial membrane, 9
Synovitis, 10, 11
  anatomy of, 16
  diagnosis of, 12, 13
  features of, 14
  gold salts for, 112
  kinds of, 15
  in psoriatic arthritis, 30
  treatment of, 20
  of wrist, 194
Syphilis, 60, 61

Talwin, 150
Tandearil; see Oxyphenbutazone
Taxes, 149
Telangiectasia, 84
Tendinitis, 156
  Achilles, 178
  of elbow, 192
"Tennis elbow," 78, 164, 192
Tenosynovitis, 51
Tension, fibrositis associated with, 78
Tests, laboratory, 135
  for aldolase, 66
  for antinuclear antibodies, 27
  B27, 34
  bacterial cultures, 51
  biopsies, 139
  blood serum chemistry tests, 137
  blood serum immunology tests, 137
  blood tests, 136, 162
  creatine phosphokinase, 66
  latex, 18
  rheumatoid factor, 18
  saving money on, 151
  sed rate, 18, 27, 34, 49, 136
  tissue-typing, 138
  for tuberculous arthritis, 53
  uric-acid test, 42
  urine, 138–139
Thomas, Lewis, 128
Thorazine, 79
Thrombocytopenia, 27
Thyroid disease, 81
Tiredness, 162–163
Toilet, problems with, 216–217
Tolectin, 21
Tolerance, drug, 116
Tolmetin (Tolectin), 104–105
Tophi, 42, 43

Tranquilizers, 150, 162
Treatment
  effectiveness of, 4
  quack, 143–145
Treatment, home, 5, 7
  for ankle pain, 180
  for bathing problems, 218
  for depression, 170
  for dizziness, 210
  for dressing difficulty, 214
  for eating difficulty, 224
  for elbow pain, 192
  for fatigue, 162
  for fever, 168
  for handle and door problems, 220
  for headache, 210
  for heel pain, 178
  for hip pain, 184
  for knee pain, 182
  for low back pain, 186
  for morning stiffness, 164
  for nausea, 206
  for neck pain, 188
  for night pain, 198
  for obesity, 172
  for pain in ball of foot, 176
  for pain after exercise, 200
  for problems opening jaws, 222
  for problems using toilet, 216
  for ringing in ears, 208
  for shoulder pain, 190
  for skin rash, 204
  for stair problems, 226
  for vomiting, 206
  for walking difficulties, 228
  for weight loss, 166
  for wrist pain, 194
Tuberculosis, 48
Tuberculous arthritis (TB)
  characteristics of, 52–53
  treatment of, 54
Tylenol (acetaminophen), 7, 81, 116
Tylenol #3, 150

Unemployment programs, 236
Urethritis, 37
Uric acid, elevated, 119
Urinalysis, 138–139
Urine tests, 24-hour, 139

Valium, 81, 105, 170

Venereal disease
  gonococcus, 51
  Reiter's syndrome, 37
  treatment of, 52
Vertebrae, cervical, 188
Vertebral disks, 71
Viral infections, 54
Vitamin D, 108
Vomiting, 206–207

Walking, 156, 184
  difficulty, 228–229
  for low back pain, 186
"Wall climbing," 191
Walsh, Jerry, 94
Water pills, 44
Wegener's granulomatosis, 86, 124
Weight control, 93, 156–157
Weight loss, 166–167
Whiplash, 79
White blood count (WBC), 136
Women
  gonococcal arthritis in, 51
  incidence of arthritis in, 17
Work
  decisions about, 91
  employment problems, 235–237
Wrist
  fusion surgery for, 132
  pain in 194–195

X-ray examination, 140–142
  cervical spine, 141
  for charcot joints, 60
  for eating difficulties, 224
  of hand, 141
  for JRA, 24
  lumbar spine, 142
  for lupus, 26
  for osteoarthritis, 58
  for polyarteritis, 86
  for polymyositis, 66
  in pseudogout, 46
  in psoriatic arthritis, 30
  in Reiter's syndrome, 38
  sacroiliac, 141
  for sacroiliac joints, 34
  saving money on, 151–152
  for scleroderma, 83
  in staphylococcus infection, 50
  in tuberculous arthritis, 53
  for weight loss, 166

Zyloprim; see Allopurinol